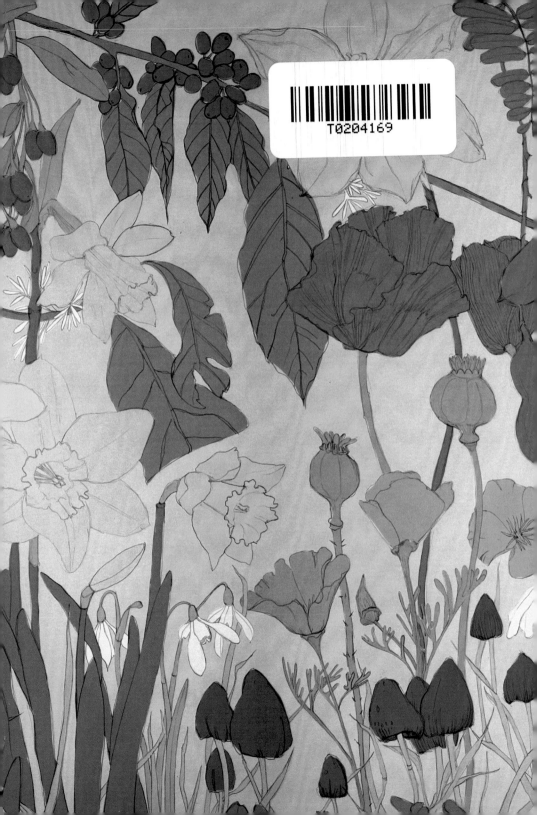

Artists Remaking Medicine

ALSO BY EMILY F. PETERS
AVAILABLE FROM PROCEDURE PRESS

Women Remaking Medicine

EMILY F. PETERS & COLLABORATORS

ARTISTS REMAKING MEDICINE

The practice of imagination and the power
to create a better healthcare future

PROCEDURE

To Lucy, who loves art and science

PROCEDURE PRESS
An imprint of Uncommon Bold
San Francisco, California
procedure.press
@procedurepress

First printing, September 2023
ISBN 979-8-218-14169-1

Library of Congress Cataloging-in-Publication Data is available upon request.

Printed in the United States of America.

ABOUT

Emily F. Peters is the founder and CEO of the healthcare brand strategy studio, Uncommon Bold, and creative director of Procedure Press. In 2016, she survived a near-fatal amniotic fluid embolism in childbirth and became an advocate for blood donation. She lives in San Francisco with her husband, daughter, and pink poodle, Benny.

This book is an anthology of interviews and features authored by Emily, paired with commissioned artworks, projects, and articles.

START

Introduction
EMILY F. PETERS

I like a simple story. It would be comforting if healthcare were all good or all bad today, if it didn't contain multitudes of moral gains and losses. It can give a person whiplash to work in the medical profession, exposed daily to the very best and worst of human nature. It is painful to be part of a structure that still produces the most expensive healthcare system in the world with the worst health outcomes of any high-income country.[1] Demoralized is the perfect word for this feeling of erosion, of "having lost your confidence, enthusiasm, and hope."[2]

The artists in this book show how that complexity, which can feel paralyzing, can also be fuel for creativity in medicine. To me, there is no one better than an artist to truthfully observe healthcare — the stories of life-saving inventions, of centuries-old professional culture, of burnout and moral fatigue, of harm — and then to use it all as material to create something vibrantly new and change our thinking.

Artists' work energizes, demonstrating just how powerful it is to share a vision for a better future. They're not just dreamers, they're people creating real change: making the sounds of a hospital less harmful, restoring agency, raising awareness of financial toxicity, fighting for beauty, repairing lost humanity, and shifting culture.

To "fight the long defeat," as co-founder of Partners in Health, Dr. Paul Farmer called it, is not easy.[3] The science fiction author Neal Stephenson explained how dystopia functionally requires less effort than hope: "It is much easier and cheaper to take the existing visual environment and degrade it than it is to create a new vision of the future from whole cloth. That's why New York keeps getting destroyed in movies: it's relatively easy to take an iconic structure like the Empire State Building or the Statue of Liberty and knock it over than it is to design a future environment from scratch."[4]

It may be easier and cheaper for us to imagine a healthcare future that continues to become more expensive, more bogged down with administrative waste, more neglectful of the humans who work and are cared for in the system. "Easier and cheaper" to imagine thankfully doesn't mean it is more likely to come true. Throughout this book, looking back at history shows us that change in medicine happens all the time. Nothing is permanent.

"What we're lacking from a little bit is the idea of what is possible," remarked Dr. Stella Safo in one of my earliest interviews. I have felt this same way many times. Writing this book and collaborating with writers, visual artists, puppeteers, musicians, architects, and futurists has shown me just what is possible.

Artists are the secret weapon. They are the way to build that "new vision of the future" for healthcare — one that is more joyful, truthful, affordable, effective, and healing for both professionals and patients. Artists shake us awake, they help us focus. Artists help us to love medicine for what it is, to be curious about how we got here, and to challenge everyone involved to a more vivid moral imagination.

It would be a much simpler story if we could just wait for a hero to save our healthcare system. Instead, it is just us — all of us — doing what we can.

1.0

TIME

HISTORIC ABUNDANCE

Art and medicine were once part of everyday life.
Can we reclaim medicine for the commons?

Early medicine was often fantastical, formed by strange ideas about illness, and containing even stranger cures. The belief that blood held the "vitality of life" led ancient Romans to treat epilepsy by drinking that which spilled from fallen gladiators. It was once fashionable to consume mummified remains for all manner of conditions, even as benign as a bruise.[1] Before the discovery of germ theory, illness was often thought to be caused by evil spirits[2] or even the result of divine punishment.[3]

Although lacking a scientific understanding of how disease was caused or spread, pre-modern societies still developed effective technologies to manage them. Medieval Europe, for example, utilized quarantine and social distancing as a public health strategy to deal with the Black Plague — an approach still recommended for dealing with present-day pandemics.[4] Traditional healers may have used unconventional language to describe bodily threats, or blamed psychological disturbances on angry ancestors, but they recognized the same maladies that haunt us in modern times.[5] Over time, as humans have evolved, so has our understanding of sickness: how we define it, how it's transmitted, the best ways to treat it. Practices like medical canni-balism have thankfully been abandoned, but some healing customs of the past are with us still — while others are worth revisiting.

Throughout this evolution, the need for healing, and therefore the demand for healers, remains unchanged by time. One might wonder what people feel called to meet this demand and what qualities might they share. No doubt, the ideal clinical prac-titioner in modern times would look much different than a healer from the ancient past, partly because humankind once held a more expansive vision of what healing could be. A healer's domain once extended far beyond a hospital or office: into holy places among ascetics praying, diviners throwing shells, and herbalists digging at forest roots.

This domain also extended into the realm of arts; at the points where art and medicine intersect, we find healing practices able to speak to our deepest fears and longings — wishes for fertility or even to avoid death. Some of the earliest sculptures made by humans are hypothesized to be medicinal fetishes. The Venus of Hohle Fels and the Venus of Willendorf (pictured here) date as far back as 36,000 years ago[6] and were believed to have been used in fertility rituals with the purpose of aiding reproductive function, thereby blending boundaries between art and healing artifacts.

The practice of medicine has never stopped inspiring art. Medical phenomena — anatomical observations or even childbirth — have been countlessly documented through artistic expressions such as plays, paintings, and poetry. Leonardo di Vinci's work, the Vitruvian Man, is an iconic example of medical illustration from pre-modern times.[7,8,9] Sometimes the artists documenting the practice of medicine were themselves doctors. Thirteenth century physician Ibn al-Nafis produced an illustrated work describing the movement of blood throughout the pulmonary system,[10] and medieval physician Andreas Vesalius published *De Humani Corporis Fabrica*,[11] a book containing groundbreaking anatomical sketches.

Further examination of the shared histories of medicine and art reveal both were relatively abundant, due to their incorporation into everyday life. Nearly every culture has socially prescribed therapeutic practices, and in the realm of cosmetics, there is clear overlap between popular artistic expression and medicine. Custom has long promoted henna (*Lawsonia inermis*) as a skin dye, often ceremoniously applied in fanciful designs to mark special occasions. While desire for social acceptance largely drives the use of henna, users also benefit from its antibacterial, antifungal, and UV protective effects.[12,13] Kohl is another ancient cosmetic that finds itself embedded in common practice and has the added benefit of protecting eyes from infection and sun damage.[14] The medical utility of engaging in an ornamental practice doesn't have to be consciously acknowledged for entire societies to benefit from their widespread use — the degree of utility alone ensures a practice's abundance.

Such utilitarianism is characteristic of African art, which often takes the form of functional tools and objects, rather than ornamental pieces intended solely for display. Scholarship has found that sub-Saharan cultures don't have a distinct word for "art,"[15] likely due to their conceptualization of utility and aesthetics as inseparable. Commonplace objects, such as baskets, smoking pipes, and pottery, are beautified, infused with meaning beyond their functional purpose

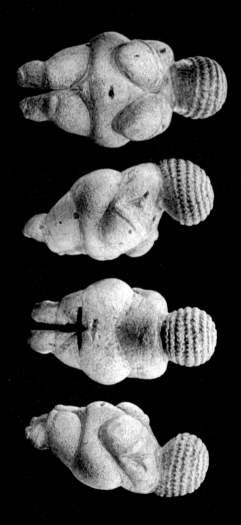

— with function expanded to include not just a practical use but a social and spiritual purpose as well. This dual purpose accounts for the abundance of art in sub-Saharan Africa, resulting in its presence in unexpected places — even the ground that her people walk upon may serve as a canvas for artistic self-expression.[16]

In societies throughout the African diaspora, medicine is also abundant and ordinary — if you know where to look. Fittingly, there exists an African American proverb that says, "to walk over the plants of the earth is to walk over medicine." It is this ubiquity, this relative accessibility, that led the art and medicine of non-Westerners to be categorized as uncivilized. Although the early 20th century saw a burgeoning interest in African art, it was still labeled as primitive[17] — even as it inspired modern artists such as Pablo Picasso. Similarly, non-Western medicine was said to lack sophistication — again, due to its reflecting the ordinary and the natural. Medicine history speaks to this duality of both holding contempt for, while relying on, the healing practices of non-Europeans. Enslaved Black healers, for example, were dismissed as superstitious, even as their medicine ways became foundational to Euro-American pharmacopeia.[18]

As capitalism gained traction under colonial rule, a new medicine model arose that disempowered the masses from practicing or accessing healthcare outside of the authority of an elite few. For this shift to occur, first the delegitimization of trusted folk healing traditions was required. Medicine had to be distanced from other realms of human experience, such as the spiritual and the artistic, in favor of a sanitized clinical approach to healing. After the French Revolution, we saw the rise of the hospital movement, which gave birth to the clinical gaze. In his essay, "The Birth of the Clinic," Michel Foucault[19] describes the clinical gaze as "a form and method of knowing that divested the patient of subjectivity and reconfigured him as a semiological field of pathological signs." He asserts that adoption of this "gaze" by 19th century doctors as something that transformed patients into "teaching and research material, objects [to] be bartered for medical progress." These hospitals, which quickly became the only acceptable training grounds for the healing arts, required their patients to be objectified by this gaze.[20] The subjective realities and individual narratives of these patients had to be generalized for clinical distance to be achieved.

Nineteenth century physician Philippe Pinel wrote in *The Clinical Training of Doctors* that making precise medical observations required reducing patient narratives to the "smallest number of facts and to the plainest data."[19] Widespread adoption of Pinel's philosophy led to the development of a medical culture that prioritized the methodical collection of orderly data and performing chemical analysis and dissection, over listening to patient narratives or nourishing patient-doctor relationships. While this disciplined approach to medicine did result in increased scientific competence, the scientization of medicine also encouraged non-therapeutic experimentation, turning the pain of patients into a spectacle.[20]

Paradoxically, despite technological advancements and efficiency gained through this reductive treatment of patients, healthcare has become a scarce commodity over the last century. This was a consequence of the industrialization of healthcare, which created an elaborate corporate structure known as the medical-industrial complex. Corporatized medicine took an especially strong hold in the United States, where the primary function of the American healthcare system evolved to prioritize profit-making over social usefulness.[21] Despite initial hopes that these changes would drive the cost of medicine down, healthcare in the U.S. now costs significantly more compared to other industrialized countries but ranks last in terms of granting access.[22] Now, those in the West still privileged to access medical care find themselves disenchanted with its emphasis on clinical detachment and mechanization and are calling for a return to more patient-centered healthcare practices.[23]

Whereas the profits-over-people model of industrialized medicine created scarcity, adopting a more human-centered approach to healthcare can increase access. Studies suggest that incorporating the humanities into medicine, as ancient healers once did, can achieve better patient health outcomes through positive shifts in our medical culture. We can look to the artistic healing traditions of the past for models of caretaking that can be carried into modern-day practice.

THEATRICAL MEDICINE

Throughout human history, traditional healers have participated in medicine theater, employing ritual use of dance, drum, and song for healing. Scholarship has long suggested these customs are more than symbolic ritual behaviors, but rather activities that led to better individual and community health through promotion of social bonding and emotional regulation. This theater could take the form of petitions to the gods for the good health of their patrons or, as in the case of ancient Egyptian healers, theater productions — complete with song and costume — to drive away a patient's sickness. In modern times, drama is being used to promote public health by bringing awareness to the harms of illegal drug use; the importance of healthy eating habits; and ways to improve self-esteem, reduce stigma associated with mental health conditions, and promote understanding of LGBTQ communities.[24] Participating in improvisational theater workshops were found to reduce mental health concerns such as social anxiety.[24]

MUSIC MEDICINE

Greek scholar Pythagoras praised the health benefits of music, while Roman philosopher Porphyry was said to have cured the sick of "psychic and somatic afflictions" with healing song.[25] During the Middle Ages, monasteries became repositories of healing knowledge: places where one could receive formalized training in monastic medicine or care in their infirmaries. Benedictine abbess Hildegard of Bingen,[25] known for penning two influential medical texts, was also a gifted musician who believed music to be essential to healing. She composed more than 70 works of "celestial harmony," including the first known opera. During this era, music became a central focus of hospitals in Europe — with patients having prescriptions for music exposure fulfilled at onsite chapels. This practice would stand the test of time: Current research shows there are numerous health benefits to music interventions, with exposure therapy being useful for pain management, sleep disorders, preventing postpartum depression, and neurological repair following a stroke.[24]

NARRATIVE MEDICINE

Participating in art can be healing to the artist as well as the observer. Many artists have found catharsis by utilizing art to narrate their relationship with illness and disability. Through self-portraiture, Frida Kahlo candidly explored the heartbreaking nature of her chronic pain,[26] while Audre Lorde penned a fearless account of her journey with breast cancer in *The Cancer Journals*.[27] As the viewer engages with an artist's work, a communion forms between them — commencing an exchange in which something is gained from listening as much as from the storytelling. The viewer's gaze provides accompaniment for the artist, while the viewer might come to understand an experience beyond their own.

The act of observing art cultivates the ability to evaluate emotional expression. It has been found that physicians gain a better understanding of a patient's symptoms after viewing drawings made by those patients.[24] Art engagement can train medical professionals to listen and to better accompany their patients in their suffering — both key to developing a more patient-centered practice.[28] It does this by teaching *narrative competence*, defined as the "ability to acknowledge, absorb, interpret, and act on the stories and plights of others."[28] A growing number of medical schools and hospitals are aiming to build narrative competence by incorporating narrative disciplines into their curriculum and practice — with offerings such as visual arts and music classes, creative writing courses, literature reading circles[28], and theater training.[24] The outcomes of skills-based art training are improvements in physician and patient communications via increased emotional recognition, empathy cultivation, intercultural understanding, and use of accessible language with their patients.[23]

SOFTENING THE CLINICAL GAZE

Doctors, who for more than 100 years were trained to gaze through a veil of detached concern, are now being asked to engage their patients on a more personal level. Their patients are rejecting the authoritative and impersonal culture that has come to dominate medicine since the onset of the hospital movement. These patients, whose perspectives are largely undervalued in our current medical system, are requesting to be treated as active agents in their healthcare. Instead of serving as medical objects on *display,* they want to feel seen: to have their individual needs be considered when patient care plans are built.[24,29] Bringing art into the therapeutic landscape creates this potential to move from viewing bodies as "medical objects" to seeing them as "events"[5] to be choreographed in collaboration between practitioner and patient.

This collaborative potential, via better patient-doctor attunement, can be achieved by instructing doctors in the arts. Art instruction can help doctors provide more compassionate patient-centered care by improving soft skills, such as their abilities to emotionally respond to patient narratives and understand their needs. Recentering human relationships in the era of corporatized healthcare will be challenging due to the ever-decreasing time that doctors are given with their patients. Art engagement by practitioners improves practitioner-patient communication and can be a solution for building therapeutic alliances in a more time-effective manner. When considering the goal of creating a patient-centered practice, the role of patient participation in art cannot be understated. There is mounting evidence to support the use of arts in managing patient care[30] also, specifically to improve healthcare outcomes — such as patients requiring less medication and needing shorter hospital stays.[31] At scale, incorporating the arts in healthcare has economic potential to save billions of dollars each year. Reducing the overall cost of healthcare is key to increasing access in America,[31] so arts engagement is a logical strategy to improve the accessibility of our healthcare system.

The movement is hopeful but slow-growing.

Art is increasingly being used in medical settings; music is being used to manage pain — just like it might have been in the time of Hildegard. Most commonly, however, the presence of art in American healthcare usually takes the form of permanent art displays (paintings or sculpture) in hospitals or care facilities[31] and is primarily accessible to a subset of patients being treated for acute or chronic health events. To transform contemporary medical culture into a human-centered one, better able to serve patient needs, therapeutically prescribed art must be available to a wider community — which requires more direct partnership between healthcare practitioners and artists. Perhaps we can follow in the footsteps of Arts on Prescription — a UK-based program that oversees patient referrals to art-related support services.[32] Maybe as a result, one day it will be commonplace for Americans to leave their doctor's office with a prescription for a night at the museum instead of a pill.

Reintegrating the arts into medical practice is one way we can reclaim medicine as a social good and restore abundance and humanity to it.

Looking Back
JAMES LEE CHIAHAN

Born in 1919, Jane Cooke Wright, MD, studied art in college[1] before pioneering chemotherapeutic agents and cancer research in her trailblazing medical career. She broke new ground by using human tissue cultures instead of lab mice while testing the effects of drugs on cancerous cells, and at the age of 33, she became the head of the Cancer Research Foundation.[2]

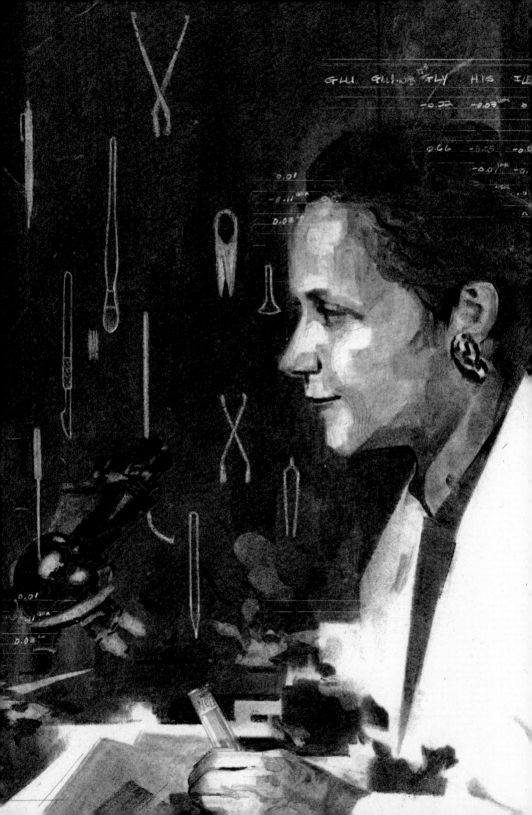

ON REMEMBERING

From a conversation with Emily F. Peters,
edited for clarity.

So much of what makes us human is tied with what we remember.

You are the person you are today because you're connected to the person you were in the past. When that connection gets broken, who are you? You are unmoored in some deep way. I didn't really appreciate how key memory is to what makes us who we are until my father lost his memory.

I also think that we suffer from a kind of hypercog-nitivism in the Western world where you're nothing unless you can think, unless you have intact cognition, unless you can be a productive member of society, unless you can remember things, unless you can add to the conversation. When you can't do these things, when you lose your memories or develop dementia, then you are treated like less of a person. Other cul-tures, particularly in the East, don't emphasize this cognitivism in the same way. Elderhood and memory loss are afforded respect, not ridicule.

Of course, memories change just like stories change. We think of memories as a reflection of how things actually happened, as correspondence, yet our memories change as we evolve; they become more a reflection of who we are today. What you remember isn't exactly what happened. You remember what you must to support the person you have become. That same thing happens with stories as you reflect on the events to create a narrative.

That's one of the reasons why I enjoy writing. Writing clarifies. It helps you understand your experience. What did this mean to me? I love telling stories: stories about myself and stories that people haven't heard about in medicine and medical history.

I found it incredibly rewarding to write about Daniel Hill Williams in my book *Heart: A History*. He was a Black man who lived in Chicago and used to work as a guitar player on river boats. He had no formal medical training until he decided he wanted to become a doctor and was employed by barber surgeons, professionals who cut hair as well as pulled teeth and performed bloodletting. He eventually went to medical school and became the first documented surgeon to operate on the human heart.

Then there were surgeons like Clarence Walton Lillehei, who literally created a human heart-lung machine by anesthetizing parents and having their blood perfuse the brain of their child undergoing open-heart surgery. I don't think courage is the right word. It's brazenness. He was also a womanizer and prosecuted in his later years for tax fraud. A real human, weak and extreme.

The first cardiac catheterization was done by Werner Forssmann on himself. The first studies of arrhythmias were done by a young Englishman who was experimenting, eventually learned the substrate for what causes rhythms in the heart, electrocuted himself, and died. There's something deeply moral about what some of these pioneering physicians and surgeons did on behalf of medical innovation and discovery. They didn't want to take on the moral responsibility to experiment and maybe harm other people, so they worked on themselves.

Those stories are amazing. They make me feel like I'm in this wonderful and intellectual tradition of storytelling. One of the reasons I was attracted to medicine in the first place was that it has such a long and rich history. In going to medical school, I was consciously joining into this historical tradition, these stories going back millennia.

Why do so many physicians write? Why do some physicians make really great writers? A lot of it has to do with how we're trained to be interested in people.

To be observant of things outside of ourselves. A large subset of physicians are very introspective people.

Your first patient, your first patient death, your first prescription, your first altercation with another colleague. Those experiences are very vivid. My experience with my father and having to remember for him also impacted my writing and storytelling. Remembering the things my father did. He grew up in poverty in rural India, doing his homework under streetlamps with borrowed books. He was an accomplished scientist who genetically modified crop plants to increase food production. Never forgetting where he came from, he devoted a large portion of his savings to creating five endowed scholarships for underprivileged undergraduate and graduate students in Fargo and on Long Island. When he could no longer do basic things, my dad didn't want to admit it. With memory loss, what's happening conflicts with how you view yourself. It creates dissonance.

My dad was still the person he was in part because I remembered what he was. I still thought of him as my father, and I still remembered the things he enjoyed. The continuity in my own mind helped him to continue to be himself. Sometimes memory becomes a burden that has to be carried by your loved ones.

My father always said, "It's not what you remember, but what others remember about you." In medicine, what we remember about our history and our own stories integrates into our views of who we are and who we want to be. What will others remember about us?

BOUNDARY SAINTS

How symbols of power and piety could
shape the future of religious hospitals.

My father-in-law — a jovial Mexican man whose hearty laugh was raspy and the top of whose head was unfamiliar to me because it was almost universally adorned with a Stetson — spent his final days as an oncology patient at Providence Little Company of Mary Medical Center in Torrance, just south of Los Angeles. We have photos of Mabel (his daughter; my wife) stretched alongside him in the bed, just *being there* as he passed.

My grandparents — Israel (who everyone called "Ulu" for reasons that are still legendary) and Lucia (whose sweetness belied the fact that her trouble-maker's soul reincarnated in my daughter) — took countless trips to the hospital beds at Dignity Health in Northridge, California, and alternated with stays at Cedars-Sinai. They visited so frequently one might think it was a hobby. In fact, our family health history reads like *Gray's Anatomy* and features congestive heart failure, cancer, diabetes, arthritis, and Tourette's.

The names of these care facilities lay plain their religious orientation. Dignity Health used to be called Catholic Healthcare West; after merging with Catholic Health Initiatives in 2019, the institution is now officially called CommonSpirit Health — a reference to 1 Corinthians 12:7: "Now to each one the manifestation of the Spirit is given for the common good."[1] Providence St. Joseph Health traces its origins back to a group of nuns on California's Redwood Coast in 1912.[2] Cedars-Sinai started in 1902 as a free tuberculosis hospital with 12 beds in a Victorian house — today its Jewish values are heralded by a Star of David displayed in the center-line of its well-known façade.[3]

More than one out of every five American hospital beds is run by a religious organization today.[4] While faith-aligned hospitals are increasing in number in the United States, the crossover among medicine, charity, and religion is hardly new.[5] "Religion and medicine have a long, intertwined, tumultuous history, going back thousands of years," writes Dr. Harold G. Koenig, Co-Director of Duke's Center for Spirituality, Theology and Health.[6] The emotional intensity of what Proudfoot and Shaver, in their seminal essay "Attribution Theory and the Psychology of Religion," call "boundary situations." These are the "anomalous experiences and events that bring people face to face with the limits of their worlds, that is, with birth, death, inexplicable suffering, or challenges to the moral code of a culture" — makes for a natural connection between the spiritual and medical.[7]

Boundary situations need not be ends or beginnings; marriage can be a boundary condition, as can a diagnosis. They are moments when we realize that tomorrow will never be the same as today, that change happens both with and without our choice (or at least the illusion of choice). They are moments when we realize we cannot always know the outcome of life's everyday undertakings, but we can be assured — restfully at times, fitfully at others — that every action has a result, and tomorrow only promises to be *interesting*. How else to explain the enveloping joy of hearing, seeing, holding a tiny infant for the first time? How else to explain the hole left behind by a death, which can never be filled except by tears and memories?

For humans, for eons, the answer to these questions has also included art. Naturally, as hubs of boundary situations, hospitals and worship sites are replete with it. The figures depicted in murals, woven into tapestries, and presiding from pedestals are holy men and women — often, saints (or their analogous icons in non-Christian religious hospitals) and even members of the clergy. However, the symbology goes further: Colors are not *just* colors. Shapes are not *just* shapes. Even if unconscious to the artist, who is a member of a particular society at a particular point in time, art is neither chosen nor created randomly. Art conveys something — and at a minimum, if nothing else, it highlights the society's priorities.

Anthropologist Robert Hefner calls the "psychosomatic reciprocity" between art and the body a "common symbolic evocation" — that is, some symbols evoke biological responses, cognitive associations, and memories as a benefit of evolution, to keep us safe and in line.[8] Symbols may inspire fear, anger, and bonds of love. What is the intended response in a healthcare context? Symbols there may inspire comfort during a moment of healthcare crisis, confidence in those who would give care, or perhaps resignation, which might make sorrowful sense in a hospital known for cancer care (i.e., "things may not work out well today, but tomorrow and the hereafter are full of promise").

Consider the Archangel Michael who, in the Abrahamic religions, is the wielder of divine strength. In addition to wings and a perpetually young, peaceful expression — standard fare for archangels — Michael is often depicted in art as sporting an armored breastplate and may be seen holding scales to weigh good versus evil or holding a sword over a subject. Michael is almost always central or oversized; combined with military garb, scales, and a consigned boyish face, the message conveys a figure worth fearing: neither angry nor vengeful, but when incited, never hesitating to execute his moral duties.

Consider alternatively Saints Francis and Anthony. As ascetics, they were admired for vowing lives of poverty to focus on spirituality, community service, and healthcare. With a message that "greed causes suffering for both the victims and the perpetrators," Saint Francis famously bore the stigmata.[9] The bandages that allegedly staunched his bleeding — a 13th century form of first aid — are on display at his cathedral in Assisi, Italy. Saint Anthony, who was born wealthy and gave away his fortune to the poor, is known as the patron saint of lost things. It is no accident that in San Francisco's Tenderloin area, a healthcare institution offering "whole person care" to a safety net community with "an emphasis on access and dignity" named itself the St. Anthony's Medical Clinic.

Will all who visit a Catholic hospital and find the figure of Saints Michael, Francis, or Anthony take in their expression and position of deference to their charge, then infer the same meaning? *Of course, no.* Will the thoughts of a visitor to Cedars-Sinai in Los Angeles, gazing upon the glass shapes in the lobby, change over time? *Of course, yes.* The ancient Greek philosopher Heraclitus of Ephesus is credited with describing *change* as life's only constant.

Religious hospitals continue to evolve their missions and morals in the modern American healthcare landscape. And they appear to be facing their own boundary situation — a time of "challenges to the moral code of a culture" and a shifting of meaning — as critical attention turns to faltering health outcomes; the toxicity of rising costs of care; and the paucity of women's healthcare instead of it being standard practice and broadly accessible. A 2017 survey found that nearly 75% of patients did not care about the religious affiliation of their hospital or health network.[10] A separate study from the same year found that one in five Catholic hospitals did not explicitly disclose their religious affiliation on their websites.[11]

Like many elements of healthcare, the exact position of religious hospitals today is murky, difficult to discern. According to *The New York Times*, in 1968, nearly every Catholic hospital had a nun or priest as the chief executive; by 2011, only eight remained.[12] There has been a steep decline in the population of American nuns who once inexpensively staffed many medical facilities under a vow of poverty. It is predicted there will be fewer than

1,000 nuns in the U.S. by 2042, with the average sister now 80 years old.[13] One recent study found that Catholic hospitals were spending less on charity care than their for-profit contemporaries.[14] Another report found some religious hospitals are being taken over by for-profit management, calling into question the bona fides of religious status for tax benefits as well as exemption from the National Labor Relations Act.[15]

Balancing healthcare against the pursuit of financial viability — let alone profitability — forces the risk of inequity, at least in our current world. We *can* do better. However, borrowing from the language of all that is good and holy, modernity's temptation to boost productivity, in the interest of supposedly raising human living standards *over here*, in exchange for *the viability of life itself* over there, results in the most diabolical of devil's bargains.

Consider California's Central Valley, where "eight counties grow about half of the nation's fruits and vegetables."[16] Just breathing there is risky amid a toxic swirl of weather, the mountainous bowl that aggregates Northern California's smoky dust, and the detritus of industry, pesticides, and millions of cows. According to *Bloomberg*, citing the World Health Organization's air quality ranking, "of the ten worst performing cities [in the United States], five are located in California's Central Valley."[17]

Emphysema, heart disease, cancer, and pediatric asthma; run-ins with tractors; car crashes on the I-5 Freeway, California Highway 99, and the rural roads that connect and extend from them all occur in the Central Valley. Such a complex collection of conditions requires a range of medical intervention capabilities, from traumatic injury response to chronic care management, across a region that is distributed both geographically and socioeconomically. Nearly half of the residents in Fresno County qualify for Medi-Cal, California's Medicaid program, yet at alternate ends of the road are Los Angeles and Sacramento, with Silicon Valley and San Francisco just a connector and a junction away.

As a result, those with the greatest need often have to travel the farthest to get a level of care advanced enough to address their ailments. Similar conditions exist across the Upper Midwest Plains States, the Deep South, the Carolinas, Vermont, Maine, Kansas, New Mexico, Upstate New York, Central Pennsylvania, and Oklahoma.

In these rural areas, religious hospitals "serve patients that others aren't; provide services others don't, in areas where others have no presence," argues the Alliance of Catholic Health Care.[17] Also in each of these places, ambulance and fire services — members of a complex ecosystem of out-of-hospital care that may be best classified as "mobile medical professionals" — serve as more than just emergency responders: They become chronically underpaid and overworked primary care clinicians-on-wheels because few local alternatives exist.

The paradoxes that plague patient care — including, tragically, that those who need care most are often the least likely to locate it nearby — force us to collectively lament the risky realities of wide socioeconomic spreads and consider the true role of these religious healthcare organizations.

***

Peering into a future where the world swears it wants to be better, the words of Scriptures themselves hold to account those who clothe themselves in the raiment of religion: *How will houses of healing redeem themselves?*

One option is to emulate the Archangel Michael: Leaning into their power, hospitals could continue rapidly growing and wielding moral influence — for better and for worse. Today, four of the 10 largest health systems in the U.S. are Catholic, including CommonSpirit and Providence, after two decades of expansion and consolidation.[5]

Or they could follow the path of poverty and charity embodied by Saints Francis and Anthony. Catholic hospitals are frequently the *only* hospitals in rural areas — where the financial strains of caring for sicker, older patients have put many independent hospitals out of business in the last decade.

Is there a third option, where the paths of humility and authority coexist? Or does our modern reality need a new model — lest its archetype be chimera... an abomination?

Many hospitals see themselves as burdened with glorious purpose. They brand themselves as havens during crises, doors ever open. Places to restore both limbs and hope, with names like *providence, dignity,* and *mercy,* and the names of people — Catholic saints, Jewish philosophers like Maimonides — whose lives of boundless self-sacrifice are worthy of emulation. *These symbols should matter.*

We know the *biology* of coming into the world — and of leaving. We don't know the *why,* how it all started, or what comes next — not for certain, anyway. All this author knows for sure is that life is *interesting.*

In the absence of more concrete answers, perhaps *where* life literally starts and stops is the perfect place to find faith during boundary moments like birth, death, and the (lack of) fairness represented by modern life's harshness. The question is, are our gilded, muraled institutions of health and wellness living up to their sacred duty?

"RELIGION, AS BOTH THE CORNER-STONE AND THE KEY-STONE OF MORALITY, MUST HAVE A MORAL ORIGIN;

SO FAR AT LEAST, THAT THE EVIDENCE
OF ITS DOCTRINES COULD NOT, LIKE
THE TRUTH OF ABSTRACT SCIENCE, BE
WHOLLY INDEPENDENT OF THE WILL."

— Samuel Taylor Coleridge, *Biographia Literaria*

2.0

BODY

ACTS OF CARE

How a rising artist is using the ephemera
of medicine to assess ever larger subjects.

Assessment is powerful. It is more than watching, observing. It is an action. It is intaking a wide variety of information, considering the state of what you see, learning, and evaluating. It is both subjective and objective. It is both expert and curious. It is seeing patterns in details large and small. In nursing protocol, assessment is always the first step.

For multidisciplinary artist Nate Lewis, assessment has always been intimately connected to his work. "A strength that I gained in nursing that allowed me to be an agile, curious thinker as an artist is my assessment skills. It's a systematic way of thinking, connecting complex layers of one system to another. As an artist I can be expansive and imaginative with that systematic thinking and make unassuming connections amongst a wider range of systems or ideas."

Today, Lewis's artwork is in wide-ranging public collections in the U.S., including the Carnegie Museum of Art, the Baltimore Museum of Art, The Studio Museum in Harlem, and the Santa Barbara Museum of Art, and also abroad in France and the U.K. In just the five years since he's worked as a full-time artist, Lewis has been profiled by *The New York Times*, toured with the Smithsonian Institution Traveling Exhibition Service, and lectured at Yale University. However, in many ways he is very much still inside the neuroscience ICU, where he worked as a critical care registered nurse.

"It was such a real time. Making my latest show, I cried a lot because so much is tied to that experience," shared Lewis. "When I was in the ICU, I realized what a special position I was in, being in the most intense times of people's lives, the most fragile times of people's lives. Dealing with the most intimate times of people's lives 12 hours a day, taking in so many worlds between each patient you're taking care of and each family member. As a healthcare practitioner, you're constantly solving problems. You have to figure things out with not a lot, sometimes. You have to connect dots all the time. You have to understand all of the different processes of the body and processes of all of the different treatments. It's real."

Lewis worked in hospitals in the Washington, D.C. area for nearly a decade, including time on the surgical intensive care and stroke units. A fourth-generation nurse, he was following in the footsteps of his father, who also worked in the ICU before becoming a nurse anesthetist. For Lewis, neuroscience critical care appealed to him as the most advanced practice of assessment possible: "With neurology, when there is imbalance or damage, there can be a change in the level or state of consciousness that sometimes feels like a change in a spiritual state. It can be intriguing and mysterious. I think they are the hardest patients to take care of in terms of assessing and detecting changes before they manifest. You can't just draw blood and know all the answers to the neurological functioning elements that are not within normal limits as you can with other systems of the body. Your assessment skills have to be sharp to pick up on slight changes in neurological functioning."

A crossroad began to gradually emerge for Lewis in response to the intensity of observing in that ICU environment. He felt himself starting to keep a distance from the patients, trying to protect himself from the empathy, the pressure of being an advocate.

"I knew it was too much of a distance for me. It felt like more work to keep that distance instead of just closing in on it. I wrote, and I prayed, daily about letting me be porous and letting me be present the best that I could in taking care of patients medically, but also emotionally. I felt anchored. I had an intuition that this was going to be some of the most important times of my life, the most important lessons of my life, and I shouldn't miss out on them. I wanted to see how those experiences of opening myself up and being porous, what that would mean — internally, spiritually, and emotionally. I don't know if it was necessarily an act of care for myself because it made things harder."

Lewis's sister Leah, an artist, encouraged him to draw after seeing some loose sketches he did while in his ICU training classes. Lewis had played with sketching red blood cells as a way to "tap into the right side of his brain" during his studies and had also taken up the violin, intrigued by the sound of the instrument. His first official art project was a series of illustrations combining organs with musical instruments that he sold as T-shirts to the general public as well as colleagues in the hospital. A favorite was "Anatomical Headphones," where vertebrae connected two cross-sections of a brain with a plug made of an external ventricular drain device used to balance a patient's intracranial pressure. The work was featured in *Scrubs Magazine,*[1] where Lewis, then just 26 years old, was quoted as saying that art "helped make me a more creative thinker and a better nurse."

Lewis was changing, working both as a nurse and an artist. With his sister, he designed an installation for the Artomatic art festival in 2012, combining the images of red blood cells and sheet music. In 2013, he created his first solo works using the paper artifacts of intimate daily life in the ICU as his canvas, the rhythms of electrocardiogram readings collaged with sheet music and images from anatomy textbooks. Lewis started scanning, enlarging, and printing the diagnostic images into larger sheets of archival paper, cutting patterns into the paper with a blade. Then, new works were sculpted into black-and-white self-portraits of his own body.

"I started making these cuts, and this alchemy happened," Lewis told the Weatherspoon Art Museum.[2] "The sheet of paper was like an organism, treating it almost like they were monuments to the patients I took care of while I was working in the ICU at that time. Working with the paper, I was thinking about all the experiences that were present, the microbiological world, the world of care, the world of genetics and in DNA, the relationships and disease process and tissue — this was all bound up in the many different textures I was bringing out within the paper. The care for the paper and that precise action — a very surgical way of approaching things."

His attention started to shift, from the bedside to assessing history, race, and politics. Lewis added photos of protests at the 2017 inauguration with the cuts in the paper. A residency with Pioneer Works in Brooklyn, New York, gave him the opportunity to leave nursing to work full-time as an artist, taking the language and visuals of medicine with him. In his subsequent "Probing the Land" series, the patient body was replaced by photos of Confederate monuments, studied as elements of anatomy and diagnostics.

"The monument pieces came from a place of an assessment, a place of understanding the temperature and status of them in the political climate — the beliefs about them in the state of conversations at the time."

In his work today, Lewis is expanding even further the scope of his assessment. Bringing in new elements of music, movement, and video, he continues to incorporate diagnostic imagery from ultrasounds, CAT scans, and angiograms, including from COVID patients during the pandemic.

"That kind of assessment imagery speaks to so many things for me," said Lewis. "It can speak to race, to class, life choices, individual choices, geographical regions, and to things that we can't particularly explain. It's dense."

In exploring the ways ultrasound is used in both diagnostic imagery on the physical body and, with Doppler radar, to evaluate the weather and climate change data, Lewis is connecting patterns of listening to our individual and climate health. From the work of "seeing with sound," he is tuning in to new systems, caring for new elements, looking for healing in ever-larger systems.

"I'm just starting to understand things, exploring within processes that are showing me other threads to continue to follow," said Lewis. "None of this would happen if I didn't live in that porous way for that chapter of my life in nursing. I'm still coming out of that clinical way of thinking, even a clinical way of making. My art came from my understanding of systems in medicine. Understanding what it is to care for something, I bring that into my practice. I think assessment can be even more an act of caring for yourself, in a very intentful way."

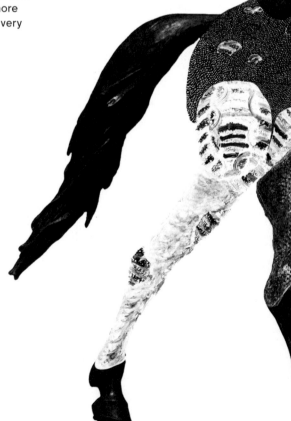

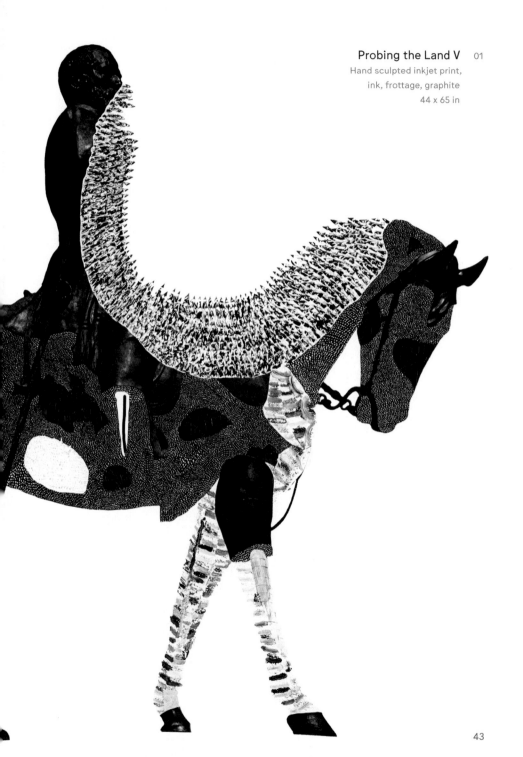

Probing the Land V 01
Hand sculpted inkjet print,
ink, frottage, graphite
44 x 65 in

02 **Still Symphony**
Hand sculpted inkjet print
24 x 18 in

03 **Orchestra in the Valley**
Hand sculpted inkjet print,
ink, frottage, graphite
70 x 44 in

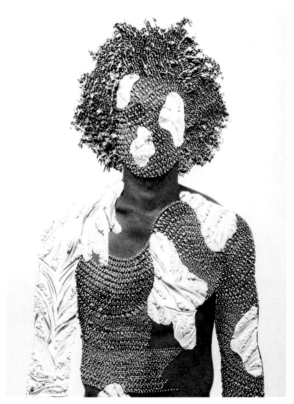

02

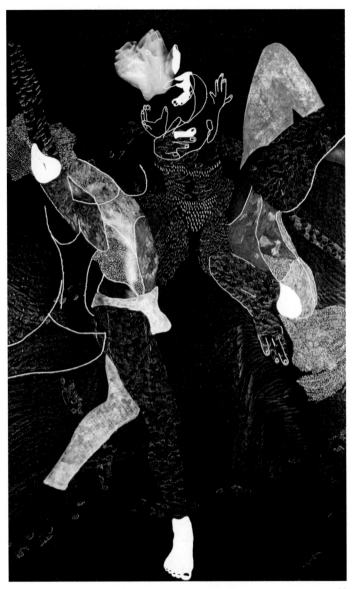

MOVING PERSPECTIVES

Discussing the lasting impact of puppetry practice
to transform the culture of medicine.

What does it look like to teach medical students to heal? To heal patients is the work, of course, but also to heal themselves, their colleagues, and maybe even the ailing healthcare system? What *could* it look like?

For interdisciplinary performing artist and health humanities scholar Marina Tsaplina, that teaching looks like movement, breath work, and culture change through the practice of puppetry animation. The 40-hour *Embodiment, Disability, and Puppetry for Health Education* program she created aims to "train the bodies of medical students and clinicians to develop the capacity for embodied attunement and deep listening."[1]

The program, which can run from a four-session module to a six-week course, focuses on embodied arts work — listening, breathing, moving, connecting imagery, memory, and emotion to breath and body — along with readings, including *There's No Algorithm for Empathy* by Hannah B. Wild, *Brilliant Imperfection: Grappling with Cure* by Eli Clare, and *In Shock* by Rana Awdish, MD, which, through the vivid experiences of her own near-fatal illness, explores "the dysfunction of disconnection" between doctors and patients.

In discovering Tsaplina's programs, Dr. Awdish recalls, "we really came together very organically because we felt the resonance in each other's work. None of that was premeditated. It was truly just valuing what the other was doing. This program is remarkable. It is also ahead of where medical training currently is."

As a conservatory-trained performing artist, Tsaplina was a Kienle Scholar in the Medical Humanities at the Penn State College of Medicine and a co-founder of the "Reimagine Medicine" program at Duke University, 2018–2020.[2] Tsaplina's work is also informed by her own experiences living with lifelong chronic illness.

Diagnosed with type 1 diabetes at just two years old, Tsaplina felt "terrified"[3] about her disability in a medical system that frames illness as being at war with her own bodymind (a term used by Disability Studies scholars and advocates to refer to the interconnected nature of mind and body). The art of puppetry gave her the tools to repair that connection with herself as well as a technique for extending the reach of those repairs.

Tsaplina's courses serve as counter-programming to the dehumanizing elements of modern medical education, within which the practices of "knowledge as possession"[4] can flourish. She describes this training as "teaching doctors how to listen for and trust the embodied knowledges of their patients."

At a time when the epidemic of burn-out among medical professionals has progressed to compassion fatigue,

moral injury, and increased suicidality, there is an urgency to equip young physicians with tools for resilience and healing connection with patients. To practice, as Tsaplina and Dr. Awdish call it, "embodied care."

Could this brief study of embodiment create lasting change in the way future physicians approach the practice of medicine? Can the art of puppetry performance help us repair the broken relationship between medicine and the body?

To find out, we invited back three cohorts of students at various stages of their careers two, three, and four years after participating in the *Embodiment, Disability, and Puppetry* training — eight medical students who at the time of the program were between their first and second years, and 19 pre-med student participants, many of whom subsequently enrolled in medical school — to share with Tsaplina and Dr. Awdish the impact of their experiences.

What follows combines excerpts from the three interviews into one conversation, edited for clarity.

ARTIST
Marina Tsaplina

MODERATOR
Rana Awdish, MD, FCCP

Philadelphia College of Osteopathic
Medicine student cohort:

Colleen Crawford	Bridgette Klein
Dakota Degenstein	Katelyn Langford
Mumta Essarani	Dhruv Patel
José Huergo	

Pre-med student cohort:

Neha Aggarwal	Margaret Gaw	Luke Sang
Beau Blass	Akeim George	Eleanor Sao
Cassia Caruth	Irene Koc	Christina Shin
Dahlia Chacon	Angus Li	Michael Shu
Karan Desai	Maria Pita	Jack Welsby
Madeline Fowler	Bryce Saba	Esther Zhang

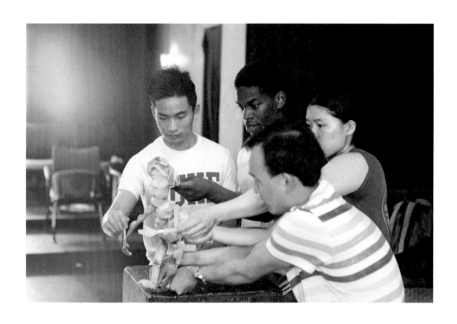

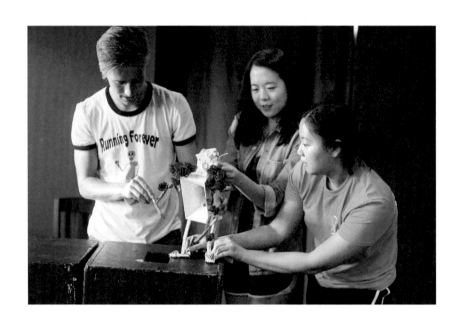

COLLEEN: In the beginning of the six weeks, I felt, "Why are we focusing so much on ourselves? This is supposed to be about patient interaction." I started to slowly realize throughout the workshops that it really did start with us. When we used the puppet or the breathwork to be still, to be silent, to be comfortable listening — our internal breath did externalize. Patients can tell when you're listening. It's not always something verbal. It is your body language or your demeanor.

BEAU: I remember how much we did during the course with "breath." We're taught very algorithmically with vital signs and specific kinds of piecemeal exam maneuvers. But being able to approach a clinical encounter from a lens of a person's breath being their embodiment in that moment...I think this attunement gives rise to an ability and intuition to say, "oh, this is where this person is right now," on a fundamental level.

DR. AWDISH: Do you feel that you listen differently when you've dropped into your body and are aware of your internal environment?

COLLEEN: Definitely. There's a certain calmness when you're in tune with your breath that shows.

KATELYN: For me, it changed my body language when I'm talking to patients. I would notice myself having my arms crossed because that was comfortable for me. This work brought me back into myself, thinking, "This is not the way I want to be portraying myself to this patient; I want to be open and able to actually listen to them."

NEHA: The puppetry practice taught me that, as a future healthcare provider, I shouldn't enter a clinic room with a rigid idea of what bodies should look like, but rather come ready to receive patient stories, to learn from their unique embodied relations with the world. That I should not come ready to fix broken parts based on abstract and subjective understandings of perfect bodies.

BRIDGETTE: I've become more aware of patients' nonverbal cues, picking up on speech patterns, and communicating their own emotions. Being able to step in when you realize there's a miscommunication or a gap in understanding. Being able to communicate more information in a way that you're sure they're understanding.

DR. AWDISH: Listening not just to what is said but how it's being said, and what the atmosphere and nonverbal cues are as well.

CHRISTINA: What's changed about how I listen is that I don't analyze. I don't analyze how people speak. I don't analyze how long it takes them to speak. I just observe more. I'm far more present now without expectations, without thinking "this is how it should go" or feeling anxious about how I should act.

DAKOTA: It taught me to be a lot more comfortable with silence, to give patients time to tell their story.

JOSÉ: Being in rotations for a year, we've been exposed to a lot of suffering. While empathy in some situations is the stereotypical, "I'm going to go in there and hear them out and let them vent," empathy can also be understanding when people don't want to talk because of their suffering. Patients are going to close themselves off, and that's okay. You can't force it. Reciprocating their desires that they want to be left alone is also listening.

"UNTIL MY OWN EXPERIENCE AS A PATIENT, I DIDN'T ALLOW MYSELF TO ENVISION AN ALTERNATIVE WHERE I WAS UNGUARDED, RECEPTIVE AND FREELY GIVING OF MYSELF.

I DIDN'T UNDERSTAND THAT OPEN CHANNELS WOULD REPLENISH MY SUPPLY OF SELF. THAT THERE WAS RECIPROCITY IN EMPATHY."

—Rana Awdish, MD, FCCP, p. 10, *In Shock*

I wish we would not underestimate how much healing can be done just by listening to someone. These non-traditional ways of healing are very profound, powerful, and cover up some of the weaknesses held by just using our contemporary approaches.

DR. AWDISH: I couldn't agree more.

JACK: After the *Embodiment, Disability and Puppetry* work, I did more volunteering in creative engagements with elders living with dementia. Trying to form these creative stories with elders was the main goal of the connection that we were forming. Intensely listening, trying to pick up on the nuances of every sentence, to read facial expressions and pauses and understand more deeply what they were meaning, not necessarily just what they were saying, getting into tune with all the small minute changes in someone's mannerisms and speech.

DR. AWDISH: What an interesting application too in patients with memory loss. Thank you.

MARIA: [As part of a cohort that participated virtually in four puppetry training modules] we received this package of disparate items that we had to put together using some instructions to create our individual puppets. I remember looking at it and being caught off guard because it felt a little bit like play, what I remember play being like as a child. Assembling something and then literally playing with it and moving it however you want and making it act on your behalf. Every time we picked it up, it felt like I'm regressing, and it felt childish in a good way.

KARAN: As the sessions went on, I was feeling like this puppet is an extension of myself. When we did the breathing exercises with the puppet or when we moved the puppet around, moved the arms around,

I thought, "I am giving a part of myself to this thing." There was some resistance initially. It allowed me to be a bit more vulnerable, having this puppet as a part of myself and that fondness growing for it.

DR. AWDISH: It is a leap of faith, isn't it? I think that's part of what I find so interesting about this work is it's learning through guided play, which we don't let ourselves do a lot, once we get to that phase of our training. It's interesting how we're taught to devalue play as something that can't bring academic learning, when that was really how we learned when we were young.

KATELYN: It also gave me a whole new level of emotional intelligence because, what the puppet was experiencing, maybe I've never experienced it. But I had to physically experience it through this puppet. I have a whole new level of gears to go through when talking to patients and seeing what they're going through.

DHRUV: During my vascular surgery rotation, a lot of patients were amputees. With the puppetry, I was able to better empathize with them and understand what they're trying to go through, in part the physical, but also emotionally and mentally.

DR. AWDISH: To think about: What might this look like? What might this feel like? And that is empathy. That's beautiful. Thank you.

AKEIM: I was tasked to change dressings for someone who had just had an abdominal surgery. I didn't think much of it. I was just changing his dressing every day, and we never talked a lot. On the last day that he was supposed to be in the hospital, I went into his room and he told me that I had been the most gentle person with his wound changes.

He said that a lot of people, they didn't care if they were using the cotton swabs a certain way, that it was causing him harm. But when I went in, I took 40 extra seconds to make sure that if he winced in pain, that I would go somewhere else and do it more gently than maybe some other people would. From what we were doing in the embodiment and puppetry work, it had been instilled in me to always be aware of how the things that I'm doing are impacting the other person and not necessarily just doing something to get it done.

DR. AWDISH: Thank you, Akeim. That is very helpful.

MUMTA: Exploring how your mind and body are connected stood out to me from the work. During my ICU rotations, a lot of the patients were intubated. When I would do a physical examination, I would make sure that I'm talking to them because I felt that they could probably hear me. Just like any patient, you are still telling them what's happening.

DR. AWDISH: Thank you for doing that. That's very meaningful to me personally.

CHRISTINA: I grew up in a family with disabilities, and this felt more familiar to me. That partnership — the clash with other team members on how you thought the puppet should breathe or how the puppet should move. "What do we do?" or "What does the puppet want to do?" There's conflicted opinions, and we're asking, "Who do we listen to?"

ELEANOR: I remember breathing with the puppet — trying to move its arms in an attempt to look like it's breathing, its shoulders go up, and its arms go out. But I couldn't figure out how to move the chest in a really natural way. I was getting frustrated because if this was an embodiment of myself, an extension of myself, then why wasn't it moving the way that I wanted it to? I remember realizing that this will happen again and again, in medicine, in times when things don't go the way you want them to, when a patient's illness suddenly takes a turn for the worse. You're not just a vessel for prescriptions and surgeries and treatments. You're a guide that guides not just their physical illness journey, but their mental and emotional and spiritual journey through this particularly difficult moment in their life.

DR. AWDISH: I hear resonance in what you're saying, Eleanor, even about disability, about not being able to make the body move in the way that you want to. Themes of inability to control, which we in medicine want to control things, and building comfort with uncertainty.

IRENE: Marina had mentioned a goal of the class was to observe without controlling, yet we're trained so much to control the situation and control a clinical encounter. I remember feeling very odd and vulnerable because what I learned was how to be in the moment with patients. There's a very physical aspect to doing puppetry that made me feel more vulnerable than in any other way. It made me think about how our patients are also vulnerable.

DR. AWDISH: It's fascinating to me, Irene, that this one experience could touch on elements of control and power and surrender, and being in the moment, and be a leveling force for vulnerability and changing the power dynamic. That's really a powerful description.

BRIDGETTE: There's a word I like, "sonder." It's the concept that everyone else has a mind that's as lively and experienced and as rich and nuanced as your own. I wish that my colleagues and other medical students would recognize that everyone is just a different version of you. To understand that it could be you, like the quote: "There, but for the grace of God, go I." Human life is so fragile, and we all have the same capacity to experience it in our own way.

I was on a pediatric hematology/oncology rotation, and I remember the physician saying to a five-year-old girl, "Just take your medicine, and everything will be okay." That's what we're up against, and we've got to change that.

DR. AWDISH: This has trained you to listen differently, even to your colleagues. Maybe things that would've gone unnoticed now trigger a response in you because they are so out of sync with fully embodied care.

COLLEEN: I want people to know that they're not alone in their frustrations of the lack of empathy in medicine. This community was really a testament for me that people do want to see change and that it is possible. We were actively working on how we can do that, not just complaining about it. We were trying to figure out how to deal with it and be the start of that change. There is a way to go about changing this.

DR. AWDISH: It feels good to be part of the solution, doesn't it? Instead of just noticing the problems. Thank you for allowing me to be part of this conversation. It's been so nurturing for me, and I have more hope in the future of medicine, meeting you all and knowing what you know.

MARINA TSAPLINA: It is a great gift to hear the lasting impact this work has had on each of you. Your words are a testament to the promise of this work fulfilling itself.

3.0

SIGHT

KATHLEEN SHEFFER 9/13/93

DATE	INPUT	OUTPUT
7/19	300 COFFEE	
	200 GATORADE	
	100 TEA	
	→ 20 MG IV LASIX PUSHED @ 9:00	
	200 WATER	500 @ 11:00
	200 GATORADE	150 @ 12:00 WITH BM
	200 WATER	100 @ 13:30 WITH BM
	200 GATORADE	
	→ 20 MG IV LASIX PUSHED @ 14:00	
	400 GATORADE	500 @ 14:50
		400 @ 16:30
		150 @ 18:45
	200 WATER	100 @ 20:30
	200 GATORADE	250 @ 23:30
7/20	→ SUPPOSITORY @ 00:00	
	200 GATORADE	100 @ 00:30 WITH BM
	300 COFFEE	250 @ 06:45 WITH BM
	200 TEA	
	200 GATORADE WITH 2× MIRALAX	
	→ 20 MG IV LASIX PUSHED @ 09:25	
		200 @ 09:50
		300 @ 10:30
	200 GATORADE	
	300 SMOOTHIE	
	200 WATER	
	→ 20 MG IV LASIX PUSHED @ 14:00	
	200 WATER	900 @ 16:45
	→ 20 MG IV LASIX PUSHED @ 19:00	
		350 @ 19:30
	→ SUPPOSITORY @ 19:50	
	200 GATORADE WITH 2× MIRALAX	
		150 @ 20:15 WITH BM
	200 TEA	
	200 WATER	
	200 GATORADE	
7/21		100 @ 00:30
	200 WATER	
	200 GATORADE WITH 2× MIRALAX	250 @ 07:50
	→ 20 MG IV LASIX PUSHED @ 08:45	
	300 COFFEE	200 @ 09:45
		400 @ 11:40
	→ MINERAL OIL ENEMA @ 12:00	
		100 @ 13:30 WITH BM
	→ 20 MG IV LASIX PUSHED @ 14:00	
	500 GATORADE	
		300 @ 15:00
	300 COFFEE	
		400 @ 17:00 WITH BM
	→ 20 IV LASIX PUSHED @ 17:50	
		400 @ 19:00

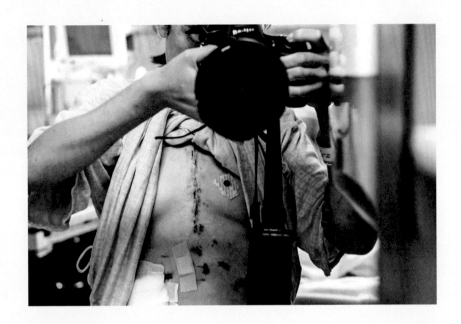

CHEST TUBES: X6.

WIRES: A x2, V x2.

PROCEDURE IN DETAIL: The patient was taken to the operating room and...

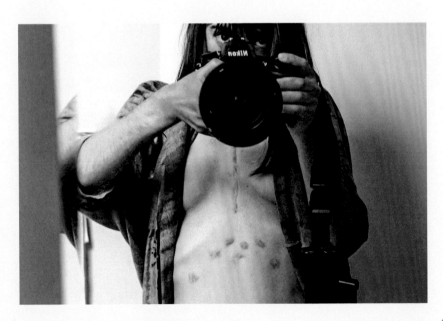

ON BEING SEEN

From a conversation with Emily F. Peters,
edited for clarity.

I remember when I met with the surgeon before my transplant, and he said, do you have any questions? I asked, "How many chest tube scars will there be?" He said, "Three." And I said, "Okay, just make sure they look cute." He just stared at me like he didn't understand what I meant, and then I woke up with six right across the center of my chest. Compare that with some people who have gotten lung transplants with female surgeons, and they put them in on the side so you can't see them. It's just such a difference to take that extra step to care about the person, to recognize that they have a life outside the operating room.

It was such a gift for myself to have photos throughout my transplant process to look back on and see the progress that I had made. I had so much brain fog after my transplant. I took notes on everything that happened so I wouldn't forget, and then took photos of those notes. It felt like everything was moving so slowly and I wasn't healing. I felt like I was in a totally different body. My progress shots were helpful to feel that I was accomplishing something in the first year. And later I could see just how quickly my body was changing and growing healthy. Now I take photos for other friends when they are fresh out of transplant, so that I can remind them later of how far they have come.

I wanted to do a project about the stories scars tell and recruited a group of transplant recipients to model for me. The goal of those photos was to take back some agency. To reclaim our own bodies. I want to show surgeons what their marks end up looking like, especially on the female body. I had so many catheter replacements over 16 years of IV therapy for pulmonary hypertension, and the places that they would put the tubes entering my six-year-old and 11-year-old and 15-year-old and 18-year-old and 22-year-old body... it seemed like they never thought about how the placement affected my self-confidence, let alone ability to dress myself.

A lot of my work as a patient, as an advocate for myself and other people, is in the small actions — my obstinacy in not putting on a hospital gown whenever I can avoid it. I want doctors and nurses to see me as a person, clothed. Growing up in and out of hospitals, it never felt right to me that the first step was to get undressed and wrap thin fabric around myself. Now as an adult with a bachelor's degree and a concentration in disability studies, I have a broader context and vocabulary with which to communicate my feelings and ask for what I need.

As soon as my chest tube wounds had healed enough, I used henna ink to outline paper cranes over each of them. I thought of it as a harmless act of rebellion, gleefully speculating what the next nurse to see them might think. The ink faded after a couple weeks, but I still see a flock of birds whenever I look in the mirror.

I can imagine being a doctor for critically ill patients and the pain of losing them all the time. I've lost so many friends over the years. I now see the doctors as human and capable of error, and I find myself wondering, have they ever seen me? There has got to be a way for us to, on both sides, see each other as human. That's what I hope the photos of our surgery scars help do.

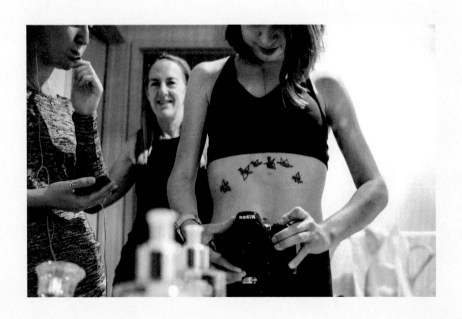

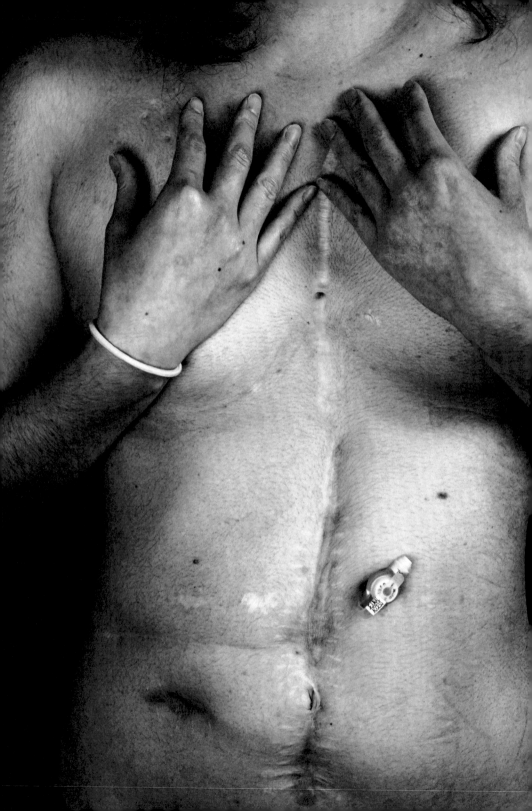

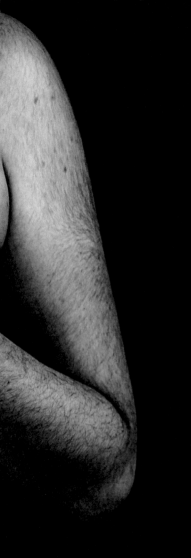

Double-Lung 01
Transplant 5.1.08
Digital photograph

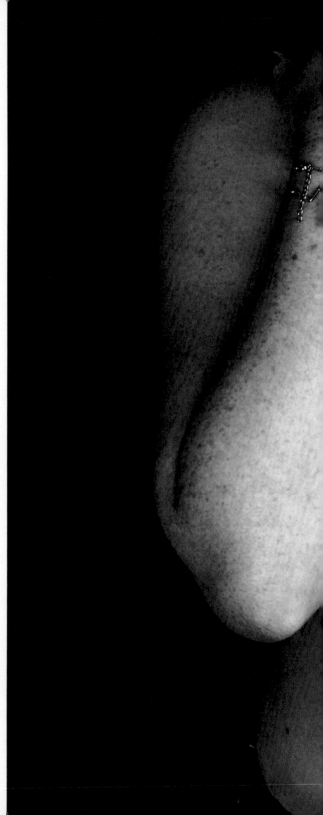

02   **Heart Transplant**
      2.3.16
      Digital photograph

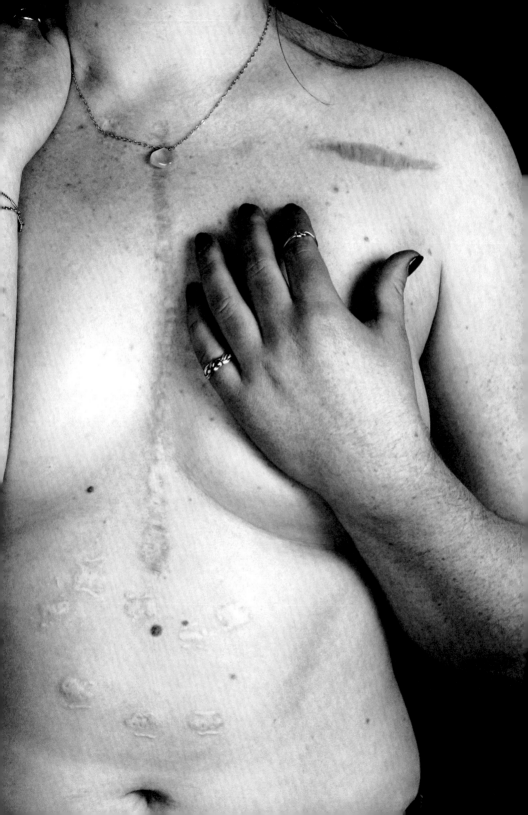

ON SEEING

From a conversation with Emily F. Peters,
edited for clarity.

As a surgical pathologist, what we see is just the human body a lot of the time. We see parts of people's bodies that have been removed, and we try to classify that part of their body to predict what's going to happen with the rest of their body. We don't usually get to see or hear the person's essence or their fears or their core values.

Street photography, for me, has always felt like a way of trying to see someone. When you pass somebody on a sidewalk, there's a whole history behind that person you don't know, and there's a whole context you don't have. A photo's incompleteness is its completeness.

When I was in medical school, people would often say: "You're never not a doctor." That is a shocking statement. I've taken a lot of effort to protect my creative side over the years. I was in bands and playing music, and all my friends were musicians and artists. I didn't talk about my music at my job as a resident physician, not because I didn't want to, but because I wanted to protect my creative life from the judgment of medical culture. It preserved that side of me, rather than let it get pushed or taken away from me.

One of the great human qualities is to want to express oneself. One of the saddest things about education, and growing up, and adulthood, is that people get this feeling pushed onto them that their self-expression isn't necessarily welcome, good enough, or relevant. Especially in medicine, these are people who've taken in a lot of education, and they've had a lot taken out of them too through the process.

Art is one of the greatest ways to feel human again. It can bring back the idea of creating something that is not for any great purpose or appreciation by others — it's simply for the fact that you're doing it.

Protect yourself from your education.

These days I feel able to talk about this more openly. I want to show younger doctors that you can be an associate professor at a large medical school and be director of services, be responsible and take on your duties, and still protect that other side of you — your creative side. You were a person long before medicine, and you'll be a person long after.

We shouldn't underestimate the power of our imagination and ideas as ideas are prototypes of reality, and in many ways they are as real as we get. This side of me has given me hope, confidence, and endless possibilities, but it has also given me more understanding, love, and empathy. It was so very worth protecting.

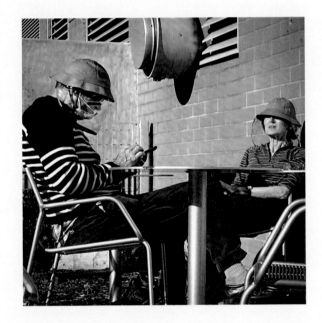

02

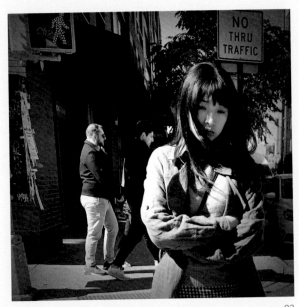

·03

4.0

SPACE

BUILDING DIGNITY

Rethinking the design of healing spaces
as community work and reformation.

What do our hospitals say about us?

If architecture "makes visible our personal and our collective aspirations as a society," as architect Michael P. Murphy, Jr. shared in his 2016 TED Talk,[1] what then is the modern hospital trying to communicate?

Is it a place of power, always expanding, with sculpture gardens from influential donors and helicopters? Is it a place closed off to its community, in a defensive posture, protecting itself first from litigation with heavy furniture and solvent-ready materials? Is it a place of crisis and trauma, surrounded by temporary tents and refrigerated trucks? Is it a place of comfort and nourishment?

A hospital "is this incredibly knotted imperfect thing, which is why designing it is such a challenging, but powerful and meaningful act. The hospital is the physical manifestation of the medical system of which we're surrendered into," said Murphy.

Murphy and the team at MASS Design Group (MASS standing for Model of Architecture Serving Society) could choose to design anything they wanted. Since the not-for-profit architecture studio first launched in 2008, they've become legendary.

They have been named Architecture Innovator of the Year by *The Wall Street Journal* and awarded the National Design Award in Architecture by the Cooper Hewitt, Smithsonian Design Museum. The ground-breaking National Memorial for Peace and Justice in Alabama? They designed that. The Rwanda Institute for Conservation Agriculture? That's their work, too.

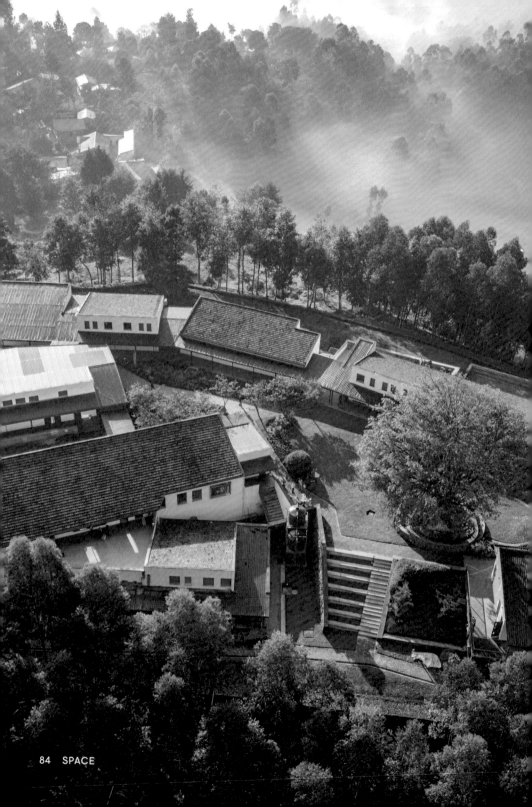

MASS is drawn to designing hospitals and medical buildings the same way that many of us choose to work in healthcare: the potential and the contradictions. In the book *The Architecture of Health: Hospital Design and the Construction of Dignity* that Murphy co-authored with Jeffrey Yasuo Mansfield, who also leads MASS's Deaf Space and Disability Justice Design Lab, they identify that tension in hospital architecture as between charity and control. "The tension between an imagined population that will need public services — charity — and the systems' overt need to shape that public's behavior so its members may attain it — control."[2] And how "architecture can both impede and advance our collective rights."

In conversation, Murphy and Mansfield expanded on these tensions built into hospitals. "The lack of beauty. The sense of pride or sense of hope. The need for authority and adaptability. These places of transition between life and death. Birth, moments of beauty and joy, moments of fear and transition. It would be too simple to just say that the hospital is an evil colonial actor, while not acknowledging that it's also saving lives quite literally. It's also not enough to say it's saving lives when not acknowledging its profoundly political and social implications on the places in which it works and operates," explored Murphy.

How does MASS approach "building to heal" within these contradictions? They start with thinking of buildings as much more than just walls and floors, but elements of the larger, complex medical system.

"The hospital is undeniably a system design. The architect is trying to use the materials that they're given to create some elegance and some logic and some simplicity in the chaos," explained Murphy. "The really elegant solutions, the brilliant thinkers, are systems designers. Florence Nightingale is a systems' thinker. She's not really designing a hospital. She's designing a medical system supported by medical nurses that she's literally creating educational programs to train and hospital standards, which are becoming policy that can be deployed across the world. She's thinking about data analysis and visualizations, she's imagining health outcomes as the ultimate end."

They remember that those systems are meant to serve humans. Through both centuries of tradition and recent academic research, we know the elements of architecture that create a healing environment: breathability of fresh air and ventilation, windows (even better — windows a patient can have control to safely open and close), clear signage, quiet, a comfortable place to sit, access to nature and beauty. Modern hospitals have often lost their way with these elements.

"I was in the ICU with my dad who went into septic shock. I was facing the end of his life and my first thought was, 'How did this place get designed this way?'" asked Murphy. "Where is the design? Has it been surrendered for all these moments of efficiency and other solutions, but somehow failed to take on the most obvious thing, which is just making experience that is comforting and nourishing?"

"Working in the medical field, we notice how the building itself often serves to stigmatize medicine and also serves to create a distrust between the medical institutions and the communities they're committed to serve. How can we rebuild the trust between these institutions and people?" said Mansfield. "We need to recognize the value and the needs of the human experience within hospitals. Not just of patients, but also of healthcare providers. How do we think about the two as collaborative within the healthcare process and what are the spaces that are needed to promote a greater sense of collaboration?"

In 2008, Murphy was invited by Dr. Paul Farmer and Partners In Health to design this kind of collaborative, human-centered, healing space for one of the poorest regions in Rwanda. With the 150-bed Butaro District Hospital, Murphy launched MASS and created a hospital without hallways, with buildings connected by open gardens and covered patios. A hospital without elevators or air conditioning, with natural airflow for infection control and natural light from large, operable windows. A hospital with bright open wards where patients and staff can watch each other and the landscape.

Perhaps most radically in the MASS approach, they aren't just designing for people, they also design with people.

In the Butaro project, that started with immersing in the community in Rwanda, listening in person to doctors, nurses, engineers, community leaders, patients, and attendants, then hiring local artisans to build using local materials, a process they now call "LoFab" for "local fabrication." More than 3,500 locals were trained and paid to excavate the building site. Local gardeners planned the landscape. Local masons assembled volcanic rock walls.

"Each context has a different set of resources, different set of tensions, a different set of trauma, or even distrust. To create a hospital or a healthcare facility that will serve the community best, what we need is to immerse, listen, and understand," shared Mansfield. "Bruce Nizeye, the engineer in Butaro, was knowledgeable on how to engage the community in the design and the building process itself, creating a sense of ownership within the community."

The MASS project in Butaro built a healing space, in a way where the process of building itself was healing. They created a hospital both physically and culturally connected to the local community, a hospital that grew to create new housing and hundreds of jobs, a hospital that breathed fresh life. They kept going, building new medical projects using those same techniques in Haiti, Liberia, Tanzania, Sudan, Malawi, Texas, and Massachusetts.

MASS Design Group created hospitals to communicate dignity.

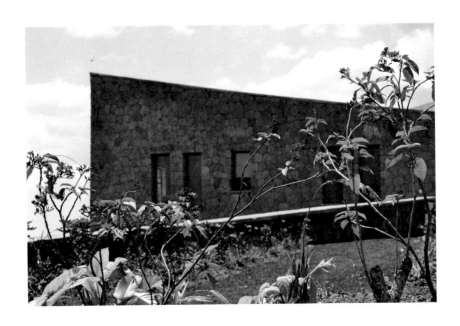

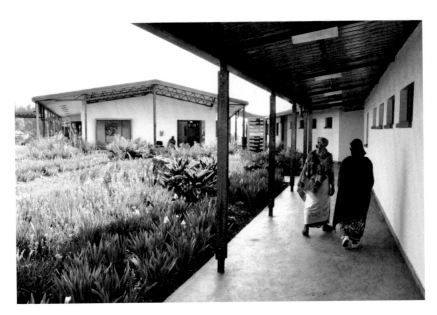

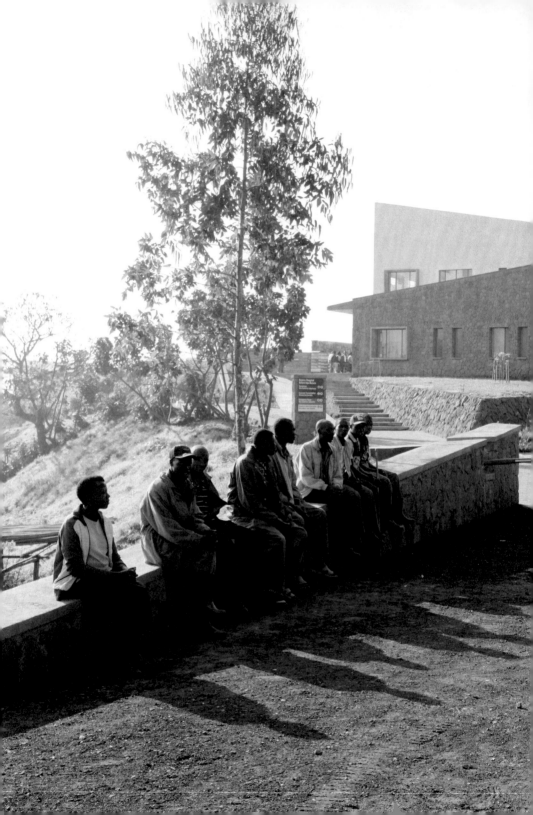

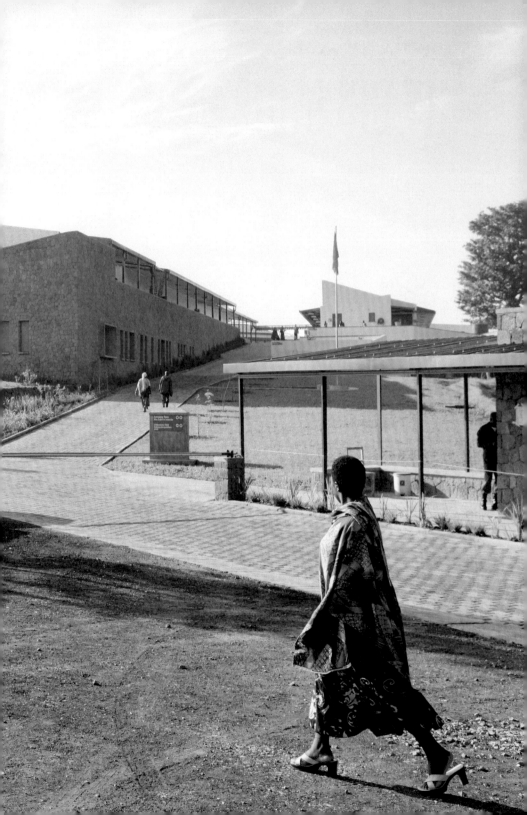

REASSEMBLY

Superstudio and radical dreaming in a broken world.

by **EMILY F. PETERS**

artwork by **LAURA J. TAFE, MD**

It was a time of unrest. In 1960s Italy, it seemed that everything had changed. Student activists were rebelling against their universities. The economy was unstable. Politics were unstable. Mustaches were large. The past was literally washing away when the Arno River flooded in November 1966, destroying millions of books and artworks.

"December 1966 witnessed the birth, from the mud of the Florence flood, of Superstudio."[1] Adolfo Natalini and Cristiano Toraldo di Francia were Superstudio's young, energetic co-founders, a brand-new architecture group that assigned themselves what *The New York Times* called "the small task of conceiving an alternative model for life on earth."[2] More than 50 years later, they still capture the world's attention without ever having made a physical building.

Superstudio was (and still is) compelling because frustration powered but never consumed them. They saw injustice clearly, and not only didn't turn their eyes from it, they put it in focus by teaming up on playful, utopian projects. Brutally honest, yet not bitter. Rejecting, and still regenerative. They were joyful, creative critics. Their relationships with each other provided a kind of tether, where they could go further out in their questioning and anger, safe knowing their colleagues would pull them back in.

Superstudio was prolific. They exhibited their work at galleries and museums, added new members, redefined categories, joined up with other artist groups, made a series of films, designed a furniture line (still in production today) — and, most famously, made collages. Collages that showed cities and mountain ranges flooded by a vast, connected grid structure, with design and nature merged in bold megastructures. As architect Bernard Tschumi told *The New York Times* in 2021, "Superstudio used the media of architecture, such as models and urban plans, to reform old ways of thinking within the profession. They would use the tools of design, but against design itself. And that was quite fascinating, because it suggested you could invent a new world with the old tools, which were the only tools we had."[3]

They were within architecture, teaching architecture at universities to new generations, and at the same time struggling with burnout from what they saw as their profession becoming boring, materialistic, and ultimately harmful to people. "If design is merely an inducement to consume, then we must reject design; if architecture is merely the codifying of bourgeois model of ownership and society, then we must reject architecture; if architecture and town planning is merely the formalisation of present unjust social divisions, then we must reject town planning and its cities," wrote Natalini[4] in 1971.

Superstudio became a close-knit family of colleagues, and often they told the story of their work together as "a diary, a travel log, records of a trip which still continues, without any illusions of a defined destination."[5] Even when on separate continents and in demanding academic roles, these colleagues constantly corresponded and confided in each other, pushing for bigger, more redefining visions. "It was above all a way of taking hold of their destiny as designers again, of rethinking it from the bottom up, reflecting on their own role in society and personal vocation," wrote architect Gabriele Mastrigli.[6]

Superstudio shows us a way to joyfully critique and dream inside the constrained systems of healthcare. To use healthcare not just to heal, but as a way of thinking about the world. In the same way that they brutally, stylishly pushed for architecture to be more, we can do the same for medicine.

We can exist as part of healthcare, while also reimagining healthcare. As insiders, we are more fully capable of seeing medicine for what it is today, where it is powerful and where it fails. The playful, protest-driven approach to architecture that Superstudio led with prototypes, immense questions, wild ideas, and theoretical focus — all created together with colleagues and friends — can inspire new work around the future of medicine. At a time when systems of healthcare are broken in so many ways, where injustice is built into the field, Superstudio invites us to adventure, to let our thick mustaches grow, to have fun creating wildly inventive new visions using the old tools of medicine, and to pull our colleagues back from despair so we can spark radical movements together.

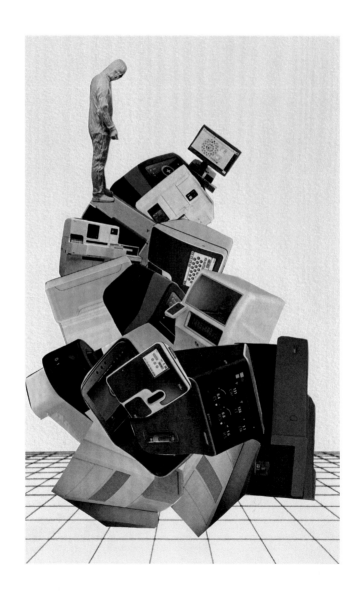

02 **Compassion**

Analog collage

9 x 11 in

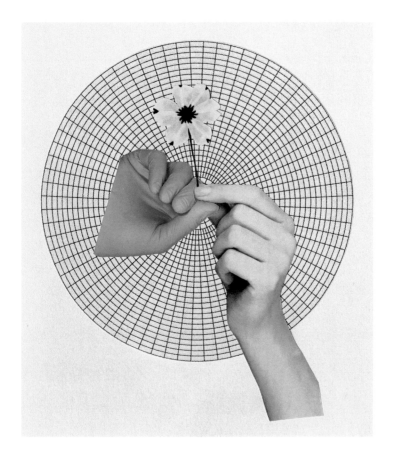

Artist Statement
LAURA J. TAFE, MD

In my work as an anatomic and molecular pathologist and as a collage artist, I love breaking things down into their basic elements and then reassembling to tell a story. It always amazes me what emerges.

When I was approached with the idea of creating collages about remaking medicine and proposed using Superstudio as a source of inspiration, I started reading about the Italian architecture collaborative. I learned that most of their work, often in collage, was ultimately out of protest, a critique of modern-day architecture. I was struck by what contemporary architect Emmanuelle Chiappone-Piriou told *The New York Times* of their influence: "Every discipline, in moments of doubt, looks back to moments in history when it has been able to reinvent itself.... What they did was regenerate architecture by asking the right questions."[3]

What are the questions that will help us to reinvent healthcare? What is not working, and also what are we really good at that we could be doing more of?

To pay homage to Superstudio, I incorporated graphs and architecture into my pieces, which are also reflective of the design elements illustrated in the MASS Design Group profile on creating architecture to heal in this chapter. Intuitively, the first collages that I made were critiques of medicine and current medical culture. I found that I needed to explore some of the challenges and crises in healthcare that I see today contributing to high rates of burnout, lack of autonomy, mental health crisis, and suicide among my colleagues before I could shift to my hopes of what can be.

In "Big Data," a figure in a biohazard suit stands on a mound of instruments, most of which could be found in a hospital clinical laboratory such as the one I work in as a pathologist. For me, this piece conveys both the power and opportunity we have with current technology to create so much data, which can be incredibly useful (laboratory test results; cancer biomarkers to direct therapy), but also can seem cold, anonymous, and overwhelming to the people who are consuming this information. While technological and computational developments are stimulating remarkable innovations in patient care, it is imperative that they are vetted and validated appropriately for clinical use in healthcare settings.

The subsequent series of three collages is my hope for the future of healthcare — areas where I see strength and where we can do even better. "Compassion" represents connection, empathy, caring, and respect — going in both directions, from the clinicians to patients and also from patient to their care teams. I recently participated in a narrative medicine workshop, and a person in one of the sessions told the story of their loved one during a hospital admission (they were receiving cancer treatment at the time) having chapstick applied to their dry, chapped lips by a nurse. That gesture stood out to them as an unbelievable act of compassion and empathy. Reflecting, they said that the nurse also deserved to receive more compassion from their patients. This story has stayed with me and principally inspired the "Compassion" collage.

"Community" brings together the architectural elements of a hospital corridor — granted, not the drab corridor that we so often imagine hospital hallways to be, but perhaps a re-envisioned passageway that welcomes and incorporates the life of nature into its space. Here, we also see children playing or discovering the world around them, the younger generation in communion with adults. As individuals who work in or engage with healthcare, building community with one another is key, and part of that is investing in the next generation. Community also means others to turn to when experiencing challenges and burnout, and collaborators to work together with to change medical culture and systems. As medical professionals, we do not always feel supported by the institutions we work for, but the human-human connections here are powerful.

Part of caring for one another also means caring for the whole person, not just our role or our job. The importance of us as multifaceted individuals is often suppressed/undervalued in the medical field. "Personhood" represents the whole people we are. We may be healthcare workers, but we are also so much more. All of these things are always with us, just not always visible to others. We carry them with us everywhere; they are our values, our pains, our loves. They make us unique individuals, and I celebrate that with this collage.

We are more than the roles we perform at our jobs. We each carry around our own stories and narratives, which are the lens through which we see and experience the world, and I argue that healthcare needs all of us, with our diverse backgrounds and stories, to continue to evolve as a profession, a public service, a society. It is meaningful to me, too, that the arch is one of the strongest structural shapes in architecture. The structure that arches over the clinicians in this collage doesn't serve as a ceiling or barrier but rather as a permeable scaffolding that holds up the entirety of what makes us individuals and allows us access to those things at all times.

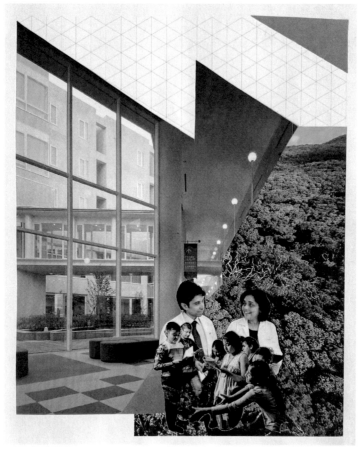

03

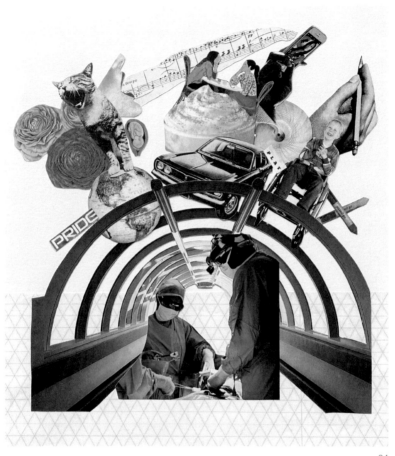

04

5.0

SOUND

TONE SHIFT

Changing the soundscape of medicine.

by **EMILY F. PETERS**

artwork by **JAMES LEE CHIAHAN**

This is a love story.

This is a love story, inside a love story, inside a love story.

To be a critical care patient is, in a way, a feeling of being loved very intensely. A team of nurses and doctors drives your body's every moment, watching you like a newborn, doing everything they can to keep you alive or holding your hand as you pass away.

To be a critical care patient is also loud. Painfully loud. Ambient noise in an ICU is about 80 decibels,[1] the volume of a leaf blower. Just one patient monitor beeps more than 45 times[1] an hour. Those who have been critical care patients or caregivers in that setting are familiar with the soundtrack to what are often the most intense days of your life.

For Yoko Sen, being a patient sounded like "People talking, screaming, and running around. Doors were getting slammed constantly. Carts rolling and squeaking. Vacuum cleaner, ice machine, call buttons, overhead speakers, televisions, people arguing. And then, all the alarms — and they're not just loud. I remember something kept beeping by my bed, pretty aggressively."[2]

As a musician, Yoko picked up the C note of one of her monitors, combining it with a high-pitched F-sharp alarm from another to make a diminished fifth, a type of dissonance so noxious that for centuries it was called a "devil's tone."

This is the story of how Yoko and Avery Sen changed those alarms and made them into a love song.

Long before Yoko Sen was in the hospital, before she met Avery, before she came to America under the official visa designation of an "alien with extraordinary abilities," she loved music. Born in Japan, she started playing piano at age three, and by eight, she aspired to be "the mayor of a city made of sound."

"I was born in Nagano but moved to more than 10 places by the time I was 10," said Yoko. "My father was a forest ecologist. I learned from his perspective that the forest has its own timeline and wisdom that is different from what we might think in a myopic timeline about cost and benefit."

As an alien with extraordinary abilities, Yoko was required to prove each year that her work as an electronic music artist was socially significant and impacting the lives of Americans in order to keep her visa.

"If I failed to prove that criteria, I would have been sent back home. At that point of my life, going back wasn't an option. My relationship with music and art making was quite a bit strained because I had to do it to survive. I wanted to have a playfulness about that and made it into a concept, identifying myself as a 'synthetic life form.' I don't think I professionally would have become the type of person I am today without the visa situation forcing me out there and requiring that my art projects had social impact."

Yoko proved herself. She performed her music at the Corcoran Gallery of Art and the Smithsonian Institution.[3] She lectured at Georgetown University and was invited as a Citizen Artist Fellow at the John F. Kennedy Center for the Performing Arts. She designed interactive sound experiences that humanized machines such as "huggy robot," where sensor suits triggered sound and video as artists hugged, and "mother tongue," where participants taught robots manners as a way to combat fear and uncertainty about singularity and to show that "we can choose our future."[4]

"I was exploring my fascination for technology. Technology as a way of helping us humans connect more meaningfully to each other and thinking of technology as an extension of nature. In Japan, spirits are believed to live in rocks and trees and in technology too, in a robot and maybe this microphone has a spirit. I always felt technology is a way to help liberate us from certain shackles of burden of history or tradition, and it is healthy."

Long before Avery was in the hospital with Yoko, before he kept bumping into her at music shows and Aikido classes, he was born and raised 10,000 miles from Japan in New York City. "My parents were divorced. So the moving around that I did was mostly from borough to borough," said Avery. "Growing up in New York City in the eighties there were art galleries, and studio spaces, and breakdance, and a lot happening on the streets."

With an equal love for arts and sciences, Avery nearly took his interest in drawing to LaGuardia High School but decided on a physics track at Bronx High School of Science instead.

From there, he continued his studies on philosophy, history of science, applied science, and technology policy at Cornell University and The George Washington University. Between his undergraduate and graduate education, Avery spent a year in Japan teaching English.

"I gained a lot of perspective being in Japan — I think among which was learning how to just shut up," said Avery. "Being an American from New York, I had an answer for everything. I think I grew when I was over there and learned to listen more and be a little bit more humble."

Avery worked surveying Japanese space technology as a Lockheed Martin Fellow for the Space Policy Institute at The George Washington University. At the National Oceanic and Atmospheric Administration, he guided executives to "imagine plausible alternative futures."

"The perspective that I got when I was in grad school, and then in my D.C. policy career, was that while innovation on the surface seems to be about technology and science — it's not. It's about people. It's about relationships. Innovation only happens because of the relationships that people have with other people."

This is a love story, after all. So, of course, Yoko and Avery met. They were both in Washington, D.C., and running into each other in "random different ways," including meditation classes and through bandmates and classmates.

"He came to one of my shows. We went to eat Korean food afterwards. We just have been together ever since," said Yoko.

***

This is a healthcare story too, after all. So, of course, then Yoko was sick.

YOKO: "Thinking in the hospital, 'wow, is this the last sound I'm going to hear' was a traumatizing experience. My memory of the time is disoriented. Lately I am remembering more about how I felt about the people who took care of me. They were nice and worked very hard."

AVERY: "I'm not as sensitive to sounds as Yoko is. My suffering was vicarious. I was the concerned husband. Wasn't it enough that she was ill and in the hospital without the compounding effect of something that was very unique to this person in terms of her musical training and because of her almost genetic predisposition to sound and being so sensitive to it. It was extra painful for her."

"My reaction was just 'let's do what we need to do while we're in the hospital and let's get the hell out. Let's just get ourselves away from the situation.'"

And then, thankfully, Yoko was well again. And that's where our story really begins.

As intensely stressful and painful as it is to be a hospital patient, there's a way that the experience draws you back. It was big, and important,

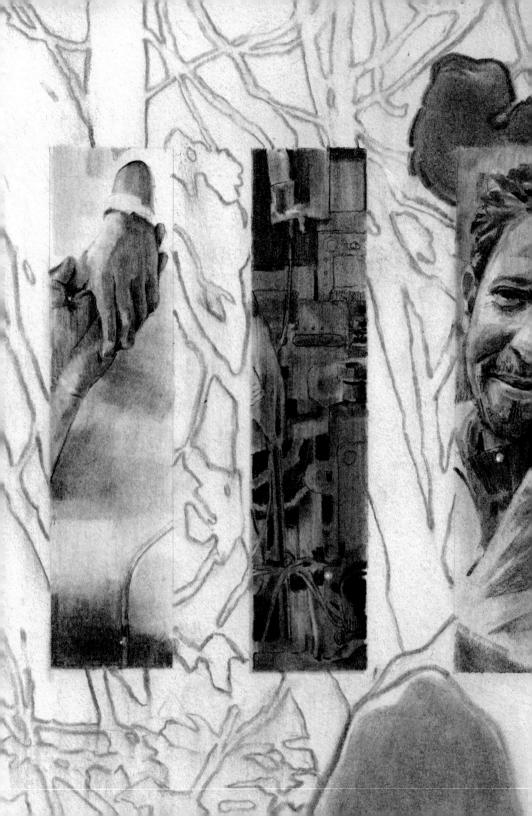

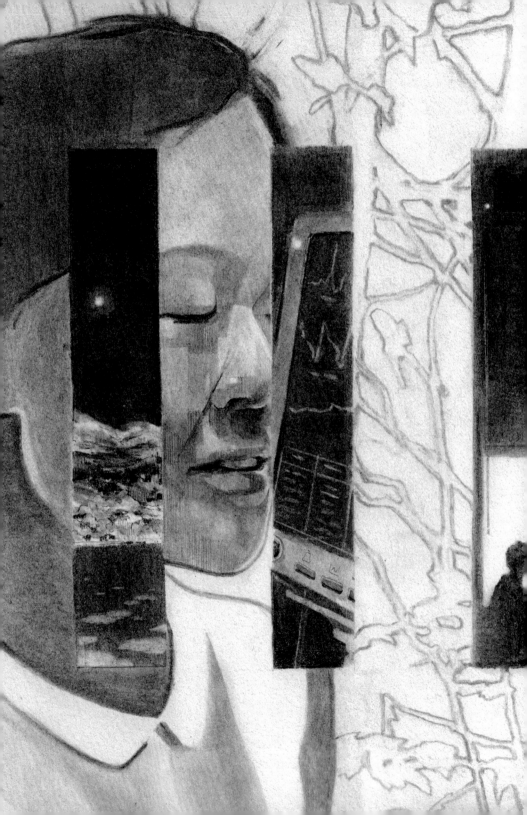

and you weren't fully present for it. You might be left curious, wanting strangely to return to the scene, even when the people closest to you were hurt by it and worked so hard to get you "the hell out."

Yoko was drawn back to her experience as a patient.

YOKO: "Learning about trauma-informed care and trauma-informed design has given me a new perspective as to how I am myself dealing with that experience using my story. If I turn that into an art project and involve people in it and make something with it, then I can sublimate that into something else. Maybe that's the reason I'm going back. I'm still processing it."

AVERY: "My reaction at first was, 'how can I remove you from this situation that's not great, but it keeps pulling you back in?' But the more time you spend in the hospital, you see the amazing humanity of the people working there, and how it is a fascinating organizational phenomenon.

It became an interesting problem to solve. It was also a way of connecting to Yoko's values. Of sound as the medium. The machine around it as the medium. The organization and how a hospital functions as the medium of this art that is also a science."

***

Yoko started working as an artist in residence at Sibley Memorial Hospital in D.C., and then with Kaiser Permanente, helping to design

healthcare experiences. She founded Sen Sound, a company that "specializes in healthcare sound innovation using human-centered design." She began sharing her story with Stanford Medicine X, TEDMED, EndWell, BBC, and *The New York Times*. And she kept going back.

And because Avery loves her, he went back, too. Right before the COVID pandemic's lockdown started, literally two weeks before, he left his work as a policy analyst and joined Sen Sound as the co-founder and research director.

Together, Yoko and Avery set off on what became a three-year journey of working with one of the biggest companies in the world to change the sound of those hospital alarms.

"We had two goals for this project," said Avery. "One was to change the sounds in the right way, but the second was to build trust and establish a relationship for making bigger changes in the future. If we made changes too drastic for the first goal, we wouldn't be able to achieve the second one."

Instead of "bold, wild, beautiful" ideas about replacing the alarms with birdsongs or windchimes, the kinds of ideas that are fun to dream up but never get implemented, they started small.

Yoko and Avery listened.

They listened to the engineers in Germany who designed the patient monitors and who surprised them by being "some of the most romantic people, really in touch with their emotions and humanity, and looking for human meaning in the work that they do." They listened to the sound in the factories making the machines. "What I didn't realize was that the people who hear those patient monitor sounds the most are the people in the factory that put it together," said Yoko. "It's constant there, more even than in the hospital."

They listened to physicians, nurses, and hospital staff, who reported that the monitors were like "a mother-in-law or a toddler or a boss who doesn't stop, an image of a fear-based, authoritarian machine trying to control you. Instead wishing it could be more like a coach, a grandparent, partner, friend, or colleague," shared Avery.

They wove those voices they heard together with data — thousands of survey points and Post-it Notes — and music (of course) to show how a patient's monitoring device could be more caring, how updating the sound of these alarms for the first time in 40 years could make the machines friendlier.

"People are willing to change, not when they are being pushed, but when they feel safe," explained Yoko. "A lot of the messaging we created was focused on making people feel safe. At the same time, as an artist, part of my job is to make people feel uncomfortable. There are moments in our presentation that could make people very defensive. We had to be very careful with that balance and respectful of the work that they had done up until that point."

The changes to the alarms were ultimately simpler than what Yoko and Avery expected. Elegant in the ways they applied their listening in the smallest adjustments possible to make the tones less abrasive.

"One of the biggest changes that we made was just make the low and medium priority alarms be less frequent. The low priority used to be every two seconds; we made it every six seconds," Yoko detailed. "With a million of these patient monitoring devices in the world, as a soundscape composition over time, that alone changes the contour of what we hear quite a bit."

The new tones are becoming available as options to clinicians in hospitals around the world, including one in Switzerland that is leading the first clinical study of their impact. In the U.S., the tones are in the final stages of FDA review. Patience with this roll-out and making the new tones optional alongside the old "is a part of moving at the speed of trust," explained Yoko.

From being inspired by the last sound someone might hear in the hospital, to three years of work creating this change, Yoko and Avery are now turning their attention to the sounds at the beginning of life and working with students early in their career. Their goal of establishing relationships that would enable greater change in the future has come true.

"Getting things implemented is, in a way, a beginning and not the end. We know that it's not like, 'Oh, these are groundbreaking sounds that are going to solve everything.' It's really not that. We are proud that we could involve people and proud that things can evolve after 40 years of not changing. Being able to do something about that, to show change is possible, for that alone, we are very grateful," said Yoko.

Imagine being in the ICU 20 years from now. Hearing these alarms on what is likely the most intense day of your life. They're gentler. They're more helpful; less aggressive. The staff is more supported by the hospital sounds and less annoyed, giving them a little more capacity to care.

Imagine the possible reach of Yoko and Avery's work. An estimated 400 million people[5] are hospitalized each year in the world. Nearly 60 million people[6] work in healthcare. A million of these monitors are beeping next to someone's bed.

"I feel very strongly that there are many different ways to make change happen. I didn't know how to do it in a way that people told me to do, so I did the way that I knew," reminisced Yoko.

Playlist
AMBER COOLEY

We've prepared a musical interlude to accompany your journey through the book. These 12 songs were hand-selected to match the themes and artists who collaborated with us. Pulling from songs with slow, soulful melodies to those with vibrant, energetic tunes, we intertwined their lyrics to form a poem.

When combined, the songs tell a powerful story: Although the path to a better future may be long and arduous, it is always worth the effort. What music inspires you to remake medicine?

Scan the barcode below with the Spotify app to access the playlist.

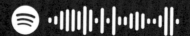

So many things are changing
I'm in a world that's breaking

The cycle continues
When we don't question what we're into

There must be a better way
Hear the music start to change

It's been a long, a long time coming
But I know a change gonna come

As every fairy tale comes real
Like multicolored flower fields

Where hate's a dream and love forever stands
All you got to do is go there

There is nothing else left holding us down
A change of key will let you out

You're not where you belong
Got to keep on keepin' on

ON MUSIC
AS MEDICINE

From a conversation with Emily F. Peters,
edited for clarity.

DR. ROSS: I am an anesthesiologist, a pain specialist, and I practice hospice and palliative medicine. One of the things that I've found throughout my career is that we don't have a whole lot to offer patients when they are sitting in front of us in the throes of deep depression, grief, or sadness.

I remember feeling helpless at times when patients would sit in front of me, having just received a terrible diagnosis, or seeing a patient on the ward in excruciating pain. That feeling of helplessness fueled my own burnout. I often felt, "What's my purpose, what's my role? I'm working as hard as I can, but I feel like a lot of what I'm doing isn't that helpful." There was no medication or procedure that I could recommend for someone who had just learned of a terminal diagnosis or whose loved one was in the final hours of life.

I became so despondent one day that I quit my job. I had to resign. I had no choice. I had to break the cycle of unfulfillment. Every time I asked myself, "What has always been meaningful to me? What are some of the things that have always kept me alive, that have always kept my spirit alive?" music kept coming back to me. One day I had the idea of offering music at the bedside to one of my cancer patients.

That interaction made all the difference. Music had been a very important part of this particular patient's life, too. He was a professional musician, and with his cancer he had lost a great deal of who he was. At the end of his life, it was clear that offering him music actually helped to reaffirm his identity, and it gave him a sense of purpose. It allowed him to die with dignity. It's because of that experience that I embarked on this mission of using music to heal.

Now I am singing at the bedside with my patients and their loved ones. Bedside singing provides opportunities for greater interpersonal connection. I gain a better understanding of who my patients are, as well as the people, places, and things that bring meaning to their lives. This connection that we share during singing helps to create a safe space for patients and their loved ones to express fears, hope, and dreams. Music has been an agent of reconciliation at the end of life, helping to mend relationships that have been strained over the years. I have also been a firsthand witness of music's unique ability to unlock memories and reaffirm the personhood of those living with dementia.

I believe in music's ability to transform doctor-patient relationships. It is heartening to see that in the U.S. healthcare industry and in other parts of the world, there's a movement to give music a presence in healing spaces.

I am encouraged by this movement, and I hope it continues to grow. I see the value that music holds to heal others and heal ourselves. We need to be filled and healed in order to be agents of healing for ourselves and others.

DR. RAJENDRAN: My story begins in India. I was a four-year-old child in 1997 when my grandmother fell sick with acute lymphoblastic leukemia. My mother and my maternal uncle would play music through the radio to mitigate my grandmother's back pain to a little extent and help her sleep. It was such a relief to us as a family. Music's therapeutic potential, the distracting potential, and ability to reduce anxiety was flabbergasting to me. My maternal uncle put me into vocal musical lessons when I was five, mainly because of witnessing music's therapeutic potential.

I started exploring the field of music therapy in the final year of medical school. In the same year, I confronted physician burnout, and I found playing veena cathartic. Music, both playing and listening, helped me cope with anxiety. It connected me to what my grandmother would have felt with music and how calming that was for her. I started advocating for the importance of integrating music into healthcare infrastructures. In any human culture, music is such an intimate part of life. While some countries have successfully included music therapy in their health-care infrastructures, with it available as an accredited professional service, many countries, despite hous-ing rich musical repertoires, have not yet ingrained music into healthcare practice.

In the past two decades, there has been growing interest around music therapy. Burgeoning research (randomized controlled trials) report music therapy's significant positive impact on several clinical ave-nues, including autistic spectrum disorders, epilepsy, neuro rehabilitation after stroke, anxiety, depression, stress, and sleep. Music therapy has been reported to reduce anxiety and enhance mood during post-operative phase recovery among breast cancer patients. Currently, insurance coverage for music therapy is limited. This coverage has the potential to reduce the financial burden on patients and their families. For this, it is crucial to have a robust evidence base through randomized controlled trials that substantiate the clinical benefits of music therapy.

Since music is associated with autobiographical memories, it should be taken into consideration that music therapy must be patient-directed and patient-selected rather than provider-selected. This not only allows the patient to be at the center of decision-making, but may also help in a better patient response.

While we wait for—and encourage—more research on music therapy, remember that it is also possible to support healing by offering music today. You can ask the patient before a procedure, "What's your favorite music? Would you like me to play that music in a certain way in the background?"

Music can be a companion to patients as well as their loved ones. I have seen myself how that particular small nudge, to offer music, can have a significant impact on somebody's quality of life.

6.0

COLOR

THE CHROMA PROJECT

by **ANNA ENGSTROM** and **EMILY F. PETERS** 6.1

Exploring the power of color for transparent,
transformative healthcare experiences.

Project Introduction
EMILY F. PETERS

There is a long history of connection to beauty in hospitals and medical spaces. The ancient Greek healing temple of Asclepeion, where Hippocrates taught on the island of Kos, featured panoramic views, tall marble pillars, and bubbling mossy springs[1] that still run today.[2] Early basilica hospitals included elaborate gilded religious altars.[3] Turn of the century western hospitals were often architectural marvels, including the art nouveau Hospital de la Santa Creu i Sant Pau in Barcelona, full of dramatic mosaics and archways, now preserved as a UNESCO World Heritage Site.[4]

In modern medicine of the past century, we've mainly lost this connection. Instead of beauty, our medical buildings turned to sterility and standardization. Hospitals became primarily white inside to show that they were clean and to ease maintenance, assembly lines for efficient birthing and dying. In the 1930s, Faber Birren emerged as a prominent authority on color theory out of Chicago and launched the trend of proper "factory setting" colors for hospitals to include soft mint green, peaches, and warm yellows.[5]

However, color itself is not the same as beauty. Just the same as surgery is not the same as health. As Birren himself believed, color is highly personal in interpretation.[6] "A color may have contradictory qualities, depending on the particular viewpoint of the observer," wrote Birren. "Reactions will differ as a person associates color with the outside world or himself."[7] Thinking that there is a "correct" beige or blue paint that can create a healing environment for every patient indulges the base paternalistic and prescriptive elements of medical culture. It limits our imagination of what might be healing to one person, distinct from all the rest.

As the avant-garde Florence Nightingale wrote in 1860, "The effect in sickness of beautiful objects, of variety of objects, and especially of brilliancy of colour, is hardly at all appreciated. Such cravings are usually called the 'fancies' of patients. And often doubtless patients have 'fancies,' as e.g. when they desire two contradictions. But much more often, their (so called) 'fancies' are the most valuable indications of what is necessary for their recovery."[8]

Early in brainstorming with Anna Engstrom for this project, it became clear that there was a different way to approach this desire for the very personal colors of healing. To connect color again to beauty, in a way that not just works within the limitations of the various regulations and financial pressures that have bleached hospitals of feeling, but also could serve to reset the power dynamics and relationships between patient, clinician, hospital, and community. By using widely available and affordable technology, it is possible to create an entirely new methodology for beauty and design in medical settings. A way to show beauty through color that is as natural, personal, and ever-changing as medicine itself.

Introduction
ANNA ENGSTROM

Color is one of the most powerful tools we have for transforming our experiences.

As a colorist painter, I love exploring the relationship of colors and its impact on us. I can feel my emotions and my energy shifting as I paint. My favorite colors are bold fluorescent yellow, orange and greens; for me they have a vibrancy to them that no other colors do. There's nothing more thrilling than opening a fresh jar of fluorescent orange and pouring it over my canvas. I can feel the energy the orange creates as I move it with a squeegee. I paint with bold, bright colors because it brings me joy, and I want to bring that joy into other people's spaces through my art.

As a user researcher and design strategist, I have spent many years listening to patients share their experiences and helping identify opportunities for healthcare to truly be a catalyst for well-being and better health outcomes.

From brand identity work, to designing healthcare clinic spaces and patients' experiences I believe color plays a key role in contributing to patients well-being. Luckily the healthcare landscape is starting to change this way, we're seeing a shift away from the traditional, sterile gray and green color choices towards warm, inviting home-like spaces bursting with colors and soft shapes. Companies like Tia and Parsley Health are among others leading the way. Patients are taking notice and are realizing they can and should expect more from their healthcare experience.

We're also seeing a shift towards a more personalized healthcare experience where care is more tailored around a patient's specific needs and preferences, where medical professionals and patients are working more collaboratively and patients can feel more in control of their healthcare journey and decisions.

At the intersection of these trends of more color expression in healthcare and more personalized medicine, is a very potent opportunity. What if we introduce color as a personal tool? Not just the static color choice of the clinic walls, a color perhaps decreed by experts to be the latest "healing" hue for all, but instead a dynamic, interactive tool for expression and communication that puts power in the hands of patients. How might this transform a patient's experiences at an individual level, change the dynamics of a healthcare organization's relationships, and even contribute to overall improved health outcomes?

I believe in a brighter and more colorful healthcare future. I believe that every healthcare system in the world should adopt color as part of their toolkit for designing patient-centered healthcare experiences.

And I believe the opportunities are endless.

This project is a window into what could be possible.

The illustrations accompanying this chapter are digital collages. The modified images included in the works are attributed in the citations on page 217.

Hypothesis

How might color help patients feel more autonomy and control over their healthcare experience?

As a patient, I felt the loss of control when I was admitted to the hospital during the last month of my second pregnancy. San Francisco had just locked down due to the COVID pandemic, and it felt like the world around me was crumbling. I had no idea what to expect from being confined to a small room in the antepartum wing of the labor and delivery floor. I was scared and felt like I had lost my choices for how I had hoped to bring our son into the world; instead, most of the decisions were made by a team of doctors monitoring me 24/7.

I was scared and lonely yet not alone. Feeling a lack of autonomy is one of the most common ways patients will describe their healthcare experience, based on my countless research interviews.

What if we could put some of that autonomy back in patients' hands through the simple invitation to choose a color?

No rules, no guidelines, no expectations, just simply giving each patient the option to choose a color. How might the choice of color provide autonomy for patients?

How might a patient's choice of color make them feel seen and heard? How might it deepen their interactions with healthcare providers? How might it even transform their healthcare environment?

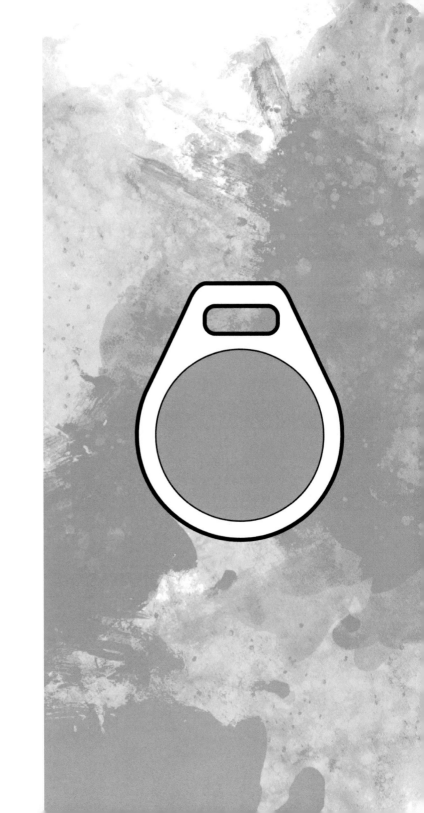

"TODAY I CHOSE ORANGE
BECAUSE IT IS UPLIFTING AND
ENERGIZING, AND I ASPIRE TO
FEEL THAT WAY."

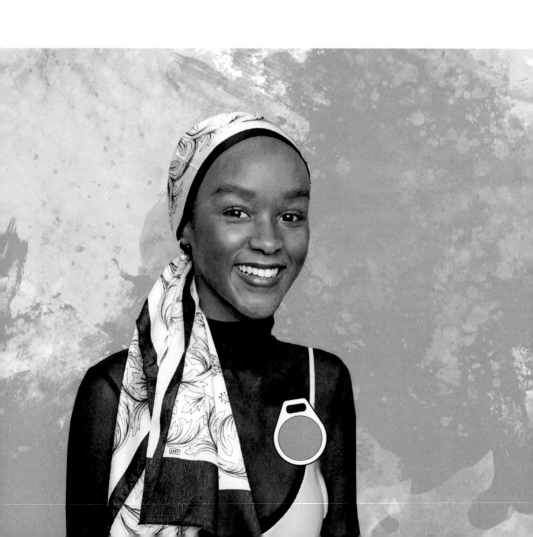

When checking into the hospital for a procedure or at the beginning of each day as an admitted patient, each patient is given the choice to select the color of their badge. The badge is worn by the patient throughout the day.

MY PATIENT EXPERIENCE:

I imagine my own choices of color would have varied across my one-month stay in the antepartum wing. I know I would have chosen colors tied to the feelings or the energy I was aspiring to feel. I needed uplifting colors that would help me feel creative, joyful, and grounded. Orange is that color to me and would have been my pick most days. I know that the act of simply getting to choose a color to set the tone for each day is something I would have looked forward to and that would have offered a sense of control.

HOW MIGHT COLOR MAKE
PATIENTS FEEL SEEN AND HEARD?

HOW MIGHT COLOR INVITE
CONNECTION AND DEEPEN OUR
CONVERSATIONS?

The choice of color on a badge is a natural conversation starter between patients and clinicians, an opportunity for the clinician to pause and ask, "I'd love to know what inspired your choice of color today?" or "Tell me about your choice of color today and what it means to you." This entry point to connect with the patient is more open-ended and humanizing than the standard "How are you feeling today?"[9]

MY PATIENT EXPERIENCE:

Many, many nurses came and went during my one-month stay, and they were my main human contact. I could only have one family member as a visitor due to the pandemic, and my husband was only able to visit a couple of times a week. Being asked about my choice of color each day certainly would have offered an opportunity to deepen the conversation and allow some space for me to share and feel seen and heard on a daily basis.

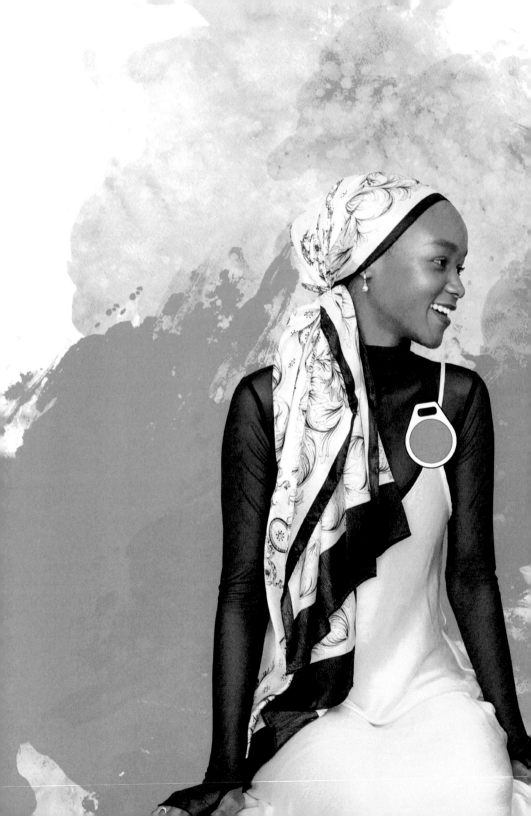

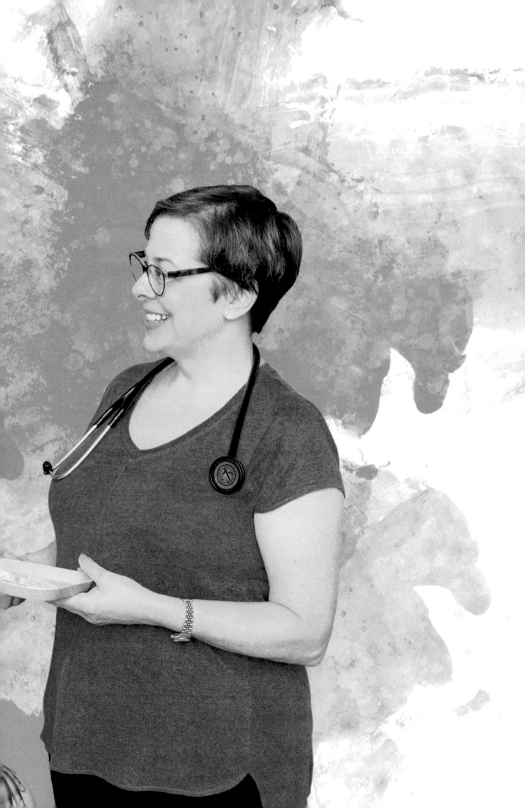

HOW MIGHT COLOR TRANSFORM A PATIENT'S ENVIRONMENT AND INVITE INTERACTION AND PLAYFULNESS?

Each badge is used as a "digital brush," allowing patients to "paint" on designated "digital canvas walls," transforming their immediate environment as they move through the facility with their selected color and "digital brush." In addition to being invited to transform their own space, patients can experience the joy and playfulness of "painting" for others to see.

MY PATIENT EXPERIENCE:

My own sterile hospital room didn't offer anything but white walls and lots of medical equipment. I was determined to make it feel more warm and inviting. I made a goal to create one painting each day to decorate my room, share with my social network, and then donate. Painting brings me so much joy; it's my creative fuel and freedom to be able to create without any boundaries, allowing me to move with my body and tune in to my senses. With a badge as my brush and walls as my canvas, I know it would have wholly, and completely, transformed my experience in that room. To have the option to start from a blank canvas and create each day or to simply enjoy the art I created would have filled me with so much joy. For someone else, it might simply mean just coloring one wall and feeling seen. No matter what the expression is, simply having the ability to transform your environment as a patient is empowerment.

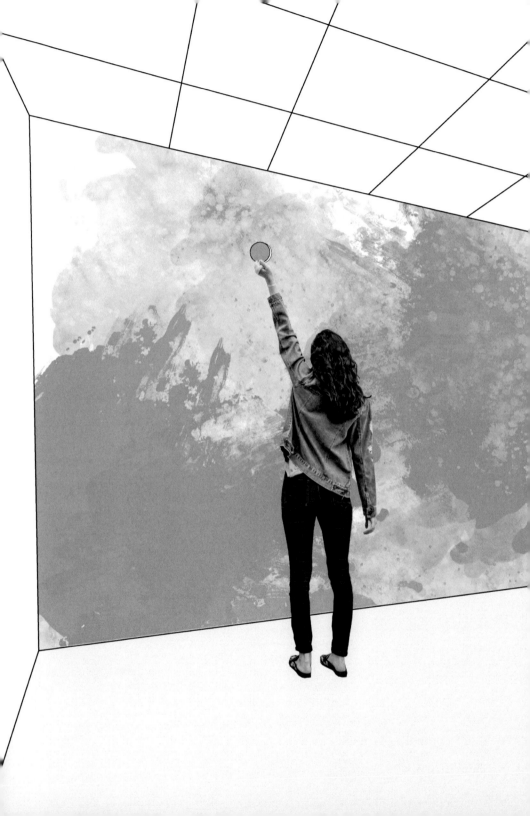

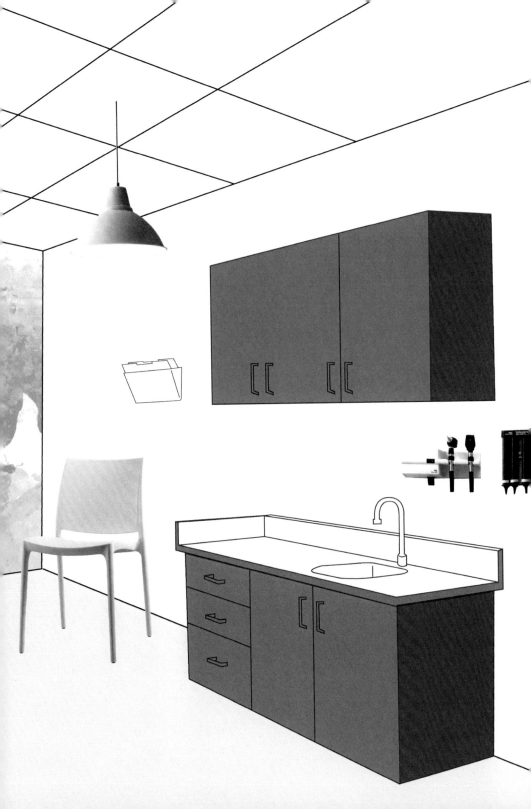

HOW MIGHT COLOR CONTRIBUTE TO A SENSE OF COMMUNITY, A SENSE OF SHARED EXPERIENCES?

As a patient, you are part of powerful shared experiences, yet rarely have the opportunity to interact with others going through the same. Modern single or double rooms have replaced larger open wards in today's hospitals, and outpatient offices are often set up to prevent infection, keeping patients more isolated and apart during their visit. Color can be used to contribute to a sense of community and be a tool for impactful expression in a way that upholds privacy and HIPAA compliance. Using personalized badges as a "digital brush," the patient is invited to contribute to communal "canvas walls" by tapping and adding a stroke/burst of their selected color. This allows patients to join shared spaces, co-create, and contribute to an art piece that is the unique reflection of the patients staying in or visiting the hospital that day, week, or month, depending on how frequently the "digital canvas wall" would reset.

MY PATIENT EXPERIENCE:

Once my son arrived at 35 weeks, he was immediately brought to the NICU. Up until this point, I had been confined to my own room with short visits to the outside garden. Now I found myself multiple times each day being pushed in a wheelchair through the long hallways between our wards. White and sterile, with carefully curated — though sparsely distributed pieces of art — these hallways added to my daily distress. If the walls, instead, had been rich variations of dynamic communal "canvases," my experience would have been different each time, inviting me to connect more deeply with my own healing while sharing my color choice of the day with others. Even more intriguing, I would be able to see and feel the colors of other patients moving through those hallways each day. It would have made me feel less lonely and instead part of something bigger, a shared experience. It would have made me curious and eager each day to see how the colors would be different from the day before.

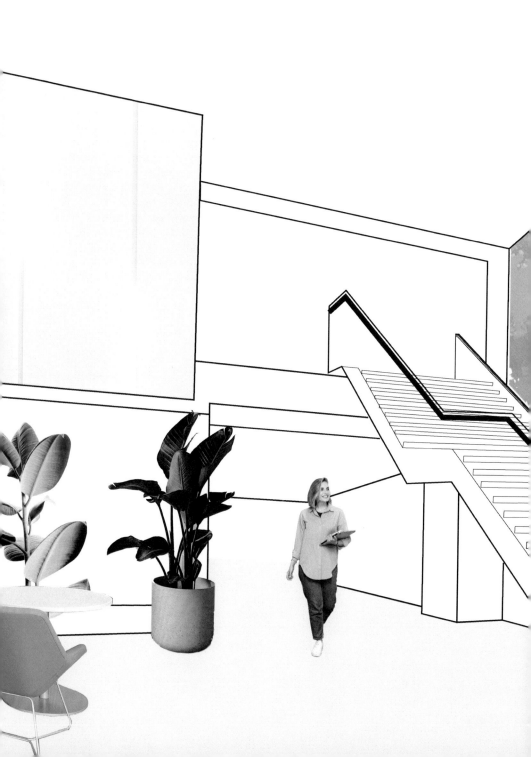

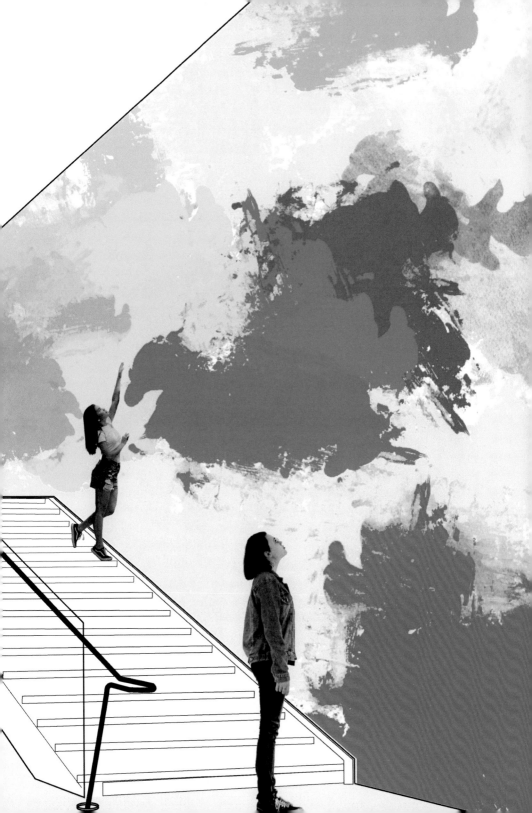

HOW MIGHT COLOR CREATE CONNECTIONS BETWEEN THE HOSPITAL AND THE SURROUNDING COMMUNITY?

From the outside, modern hospitals can be seen as a fortress, not communicating what's happening inside beyond the occasional transit of helicopters or ambulances. While they're a cornerstone of any city, the local hospital often lacks a connection with their surrounding community and, all too often today, that builds distrust. The previous concept of communal art created by patients inside the hospital, reflecting their color choices and unique composition of colors, can also be displayed on the outside of the hospital in many different ways. This offers a dynamic element, showing that hospitals are truly living, breathing buildings that are constantly changing with the people who move through, stay, and work there.

MY PATIENT EXPERIENCE:

I was fortunate to have a large window in my hospital room. Across the road was a modern apartment complex where I could observe people going about their lives. It was just a small glimpse to the outside, the bustling city around me, but it offered me a sense of connection and a feeling of being part of the community. I would have enjoyed contributing to a community art wall on the facade of the hospital for those neighbors to feel connected to us living inside the hospital. I would have liked the feeling of being part of a dynamic building filled with people coming and going, reflective of the life-changing transition happening during this moment while being part of a bigger moment in time for both San Francisco and myself — represented on the facade through my choice of color that day. Maybe a friend of mine would drive by and think, "That orange stroke right there might just be from Anna."

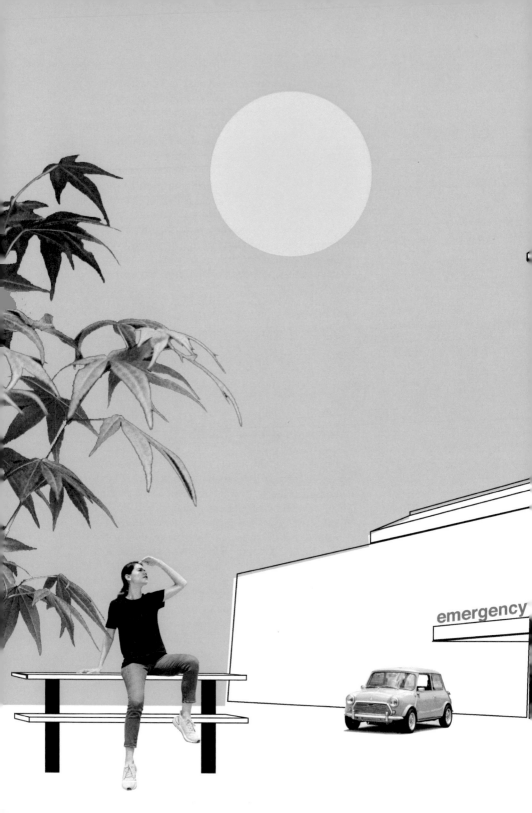

emergency

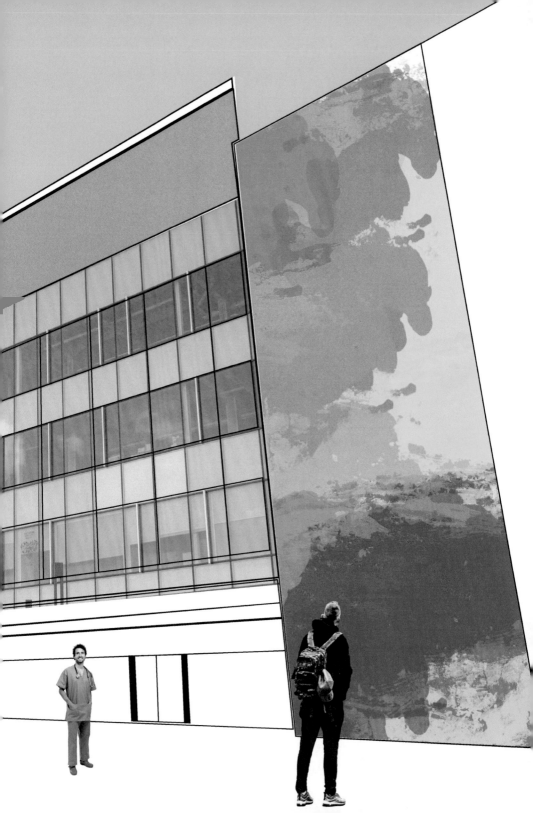

PATHOLOGY OF
MEDICAL COLORS

Everything once chosen can be chosen again.

PILL BOTTLE ORANGE

The iconic amber color of the modern prescription pill bottle is inspired by turn-of-the-century glass used for medications and comes from a specialized plastic designed to resist UV light. Not usually recyclable,[1] these bottles are widespread for more than 4 billion[2] U.S. prescriptions filled each year.

C 2, M 43, Y 100, K 0

RED CROSS/CRESCENT RED

From the inverted Swiss flag,[3] which originated from 12th century battle markers. The red cross on white symbol was adopted by the Geneva Convention in 1864 to protect medical resources from military attack.[4] The American Red Cross and Johnson & Johnson both began using the red cross symbol in the 1880s, eventually leading to a 2007 lawsuit[5] settled out of court.

C 0, M 100, Y 100, K 0

BANDAGE BEIGE

Band-Aids were invented in New Jersey in the 1920s by Johnson & Johnson employee Earle Dickson for his wife Josephine, who frequently cut and burned herself while cooking.[6] During the Black Lives Matter movement 100 years later, Band-Aid finally announced making "a range of bandages in light, medium, and deep shades of Brown and Black skin tones that embrace the beauty of diverse skin."[7]

C 5, M 22, Y 36, K 0

MEDEGEN DUSTY ROSE

Why are so many hospital bedpans, water pitchers, and emesis basins this specific dusty rose color? Look no further than Gallaway (population 720), Tennessee-based Medegen Medical Products,[8] the "largest provider of patient products in the marketplace."

C 17, M 42, Y 30, K 0

VIAGRA BLUE

Famously known as "the little blue pill," Pfizer's Viagra is one of the most identifiably branded medications on the market.[9] Originally created as a blood pressure treatment, the medication's sexual side effects, combined with the loosening of FDA regulations on consumer advertising, turned it into a $2 billion a year blockbuster at its peak in 2012.[10]

C 77, M 56, Y 0, K 0

EHR BLUE

This specific blue is pulled from the Epic standard dashboard,[11] the EHR holding records for 250 million people.[12] Similarly "safe" blue tones are used with healthcare brands including Pfizer, Roche, Blue Cross Blue Shield, Cigna, McKesson, and Virta.

C 57, M 9, Y 0, K 0

SPINACH GREEN

Green came into modern healthcare from San Francisco surgeon Harry Sherman in 1914, who found the traditional "sterile" white was too glaring on his eyes during procedures. He chose spinach green for the operating room walls, floors, sheets, and towels after trying black and other shades.[13, 14]

C 72, M 35, Y 86, K 23

MISTY GREEN

Influential Chicago color consultant Faber Birren brought misty green into healthcare design, decor, and devices starting in the 1930s. "Green is one of the best of all hues...fresh in appearance and slightly passive in quality."[15]

C 26, M 0, Y 24, K 0

SURGICAL MASK TEAL

A light teal color that will surely be remembered as essential to the COVID pandemic experience, along with other disposable PPE that were initially so scarce and then a battleground in America's culture wars. The mask design is teal on the waterproof outside and white on the inside to denote the right way to wear the filter.[16]

C 26, M 0, Y 11, K 0

NITRILE GLOVE PURPLE

Nitrile disposable gloves were patented in 1991 by Neil Tillotson and Luc DeBecker as a more durable and less allergenic alternative to latex. The purple color was introduced to distinguish the new gloves from the old. In 1992, OSHA set rules requiring personal protective equipment (PPE), including gloves for healthcare workers during concerns about the HIV crisis. By 2002, a single hospital was using about 1.75 million pairs of gloves a year.[17]

C 68, M 68, Y 0, K 0

20TH CENTURY WHITE

Before 1900, American and European physicians wore formal black, the same as clergy. Black fabric was difficult to produce with natural wood tanin dyes and for centuries was a color of the elite and powerful.[18]

Medicine went through a period of rapid scientific reform at the end of the 19th century with emerging understanding of bacteria, disease, and biomedicine.[19] By 1915, the uniform for nursing order nuns as well as surgeons (and later physicians) turned white to signify purity and cleanliness against germs.[20]

The "white coat ceremony" in medical education emerged as tradition 75 years later. Norma F. Wagoner, Dean of Students at University of Chicago's Pritzker School of Medicine, formalized the ceremony in 1989 as a way to encourage medical students to dress more professionally around patients after a professor complained.[20]

C 0, M 0, Y 0, K 0

7.0

DREAMS

RESTORATIVE

Indigenous knowledge and land-based healing
in the time of desertification.

On a dusty road in a residential neighborhood of Pueblo, Colorado, lies a garden with hundreds of cactus blossoms, and bees humming around. Today a thriving gardenscape, the land looked very different when it was purchased by April Bojorquez and Matthew Garcia in 2016.

"The land was like concrete; we had to use a jack-hammer to dig holes in it," reflected Bojorquez. The fieldsite is not just a garden project. It is an artistic endeavor and cultural space meant to revitalize Indigenous dryland ecosystems and engage commu-nity members in desert food systems and practices. "Land-based work [often means] looking at the land as a blank canvas, and we wanted to rethink that. We wanted to engage the land," Bojorquez emphasized. "Generations of people living here have a relationship with the land, people who are often marginalized [and] displaced."

In the U.S., Indigenous peoples' relationship to the land is deeply political. Indigenous connections to the land have been violently and intentionally ruptured by colonization, warfare, forced assimilation, residential schools, climate change, and the creation of borders.

Yet land is intrinsically tied to Indigenous identity. It is where we collect our traditional food and medicines. It is where we practice religious ceremonies. It is how we assert our nationhood and sovereignty. It's also linked to improved health: research suggests that access to traditional foods decreases nutrition-based ailments and that connection to nature posi-tively impacts Indigenous peoples' mental health and resilience.[1,2]

Artists like Bojorquez are grappling with this tension: land as a site of politics and exploitation and land as a site of revitalization and knowledge creation.

In Colorado, the interdisciplinary, land-based art collaborative called DesertArtLAB where Bojorquez serves as Director of Programs and Food Practice is re-creating Indigenous desert landscapes to connect people to dryland food systems. In New Mexico, painter Mallery Quetawki uses art as a form of bidirectional communication between Native communities and academic researchers addressing the health and environmental impacts of abandoned uranium mines.

Though they use different media, DesertArtLAB and Quetawki work toward common goals: centering Indigenous knowledge, centering land-based relationships, and confronting the impacts of colonialism head-on to rebuild and reimagine healthy, thriving communities.

FOOD FOR THE PEOPLE

Hundreds of millions of people across the globe are being impacted by a process called desertification.[3] Man-made climate change has exacerbated the process, and many arid regions are experiencing increased droughts and soil erosion and decreased plant productivity. Desertification is one of the issues the DesertArtLAB fieldsite is working to explore and mitigate.

Neighbors in the surrounding residential area were hesitant about their plans for the garden project. Bojorquez and Garcia didn't want to use outside irrigation, and instead rely solely on naturally occurring precipitation. To many, the plot simply wasn't hospitable land. But they knew it was possible. "Our families have been living sustainably in this region for a long time," Bojorquez, who is Chicana, emphasized.

Today, their work creates space for conversation and multigenerational, bidirectional learning. They host

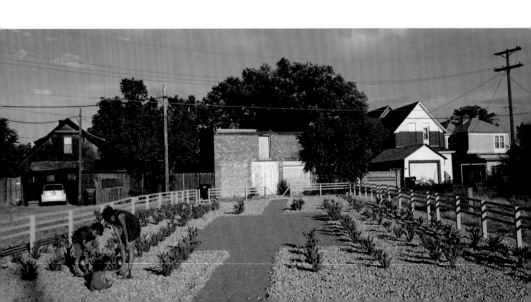

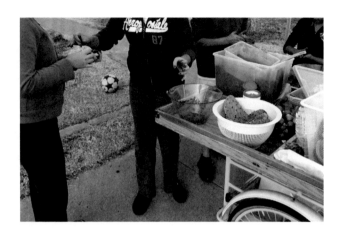

workshops on topics such as heritage seeds and how to prepare and eat cactus; are creating a cookbook with strategies for living in a drier and hotter world (the theme of the book is "don't panic, eat"); and manage a vendor bike cart outfitted to bring food and ecology workshops street-side — a mobile ecostudio.

"We've taken our bike cart, and kids will come out thinking we're selling candy, but we're doing a food workshop on cactus or restorative seed mixes," says Bojorquez. For some people, these foods are completely new. For others, they grew up eating desert foods and may jump in and teach Bojorquez and Garcia. "Some of the youth we work with are reluctant to admit they eat cactus, [but] by the time we're done with the presentation they're like 'Oh yeah we eat that every day,'" Bojorquez jokes. "Once they're given context,

[they] think it's amazing and important and sustainable."

Bojorquez and Garcia are interested in reconnecting people to the land their ancestors have long been connected to, and also in creating new and innovative ways to engage with the land. Instead of eating cactus in chili or with tacos, for example, they may use it to make sorbet. In summer 2021, they collaborated with a local choreographer, Sara Roybal from Grupo Folklórico del Pueblo, to create a yucca planting dance. This dance was both an opportunity to rethink the planting process as well as craft new ceremonies and cultural practices. "It's not just about regrowing the eco-logical system, but everything that is associated with that: re-creating con-nections between ecological systems, cultural practice, and food practice," Bojorquez reflected.

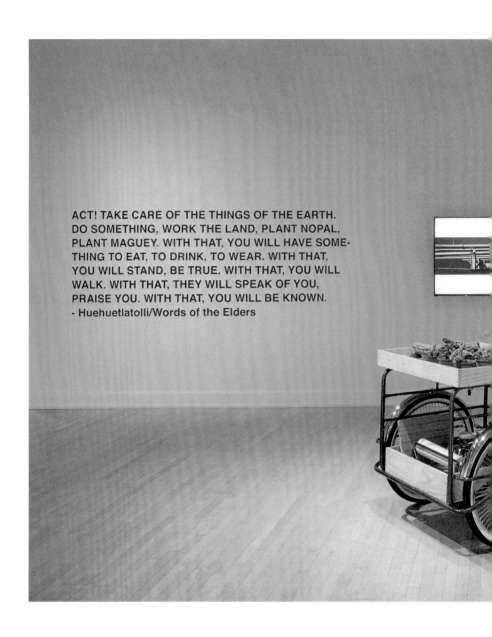

ACT! TAKE CARE OF THE THINGS OF THE EARTH.
DO SOMETHING, WORK THE LAND, PLANT NOPAL,
PLANT MAGUEY. WITH THAT, YOU WILL HAVE SOME-
THING TO EAT, TO DRINK, TO WEAR. WITH THAT,
YOU WILL STAND, BE TRUE. WITH THAT, YOU WILL
WALK. WITH THAT, THEY WILL SPEAK OF YOU,
PRAISE YOU. WITH THAT, YOU WILL BE KNOWN.
- Huehuetlatolli/Words of the Elders

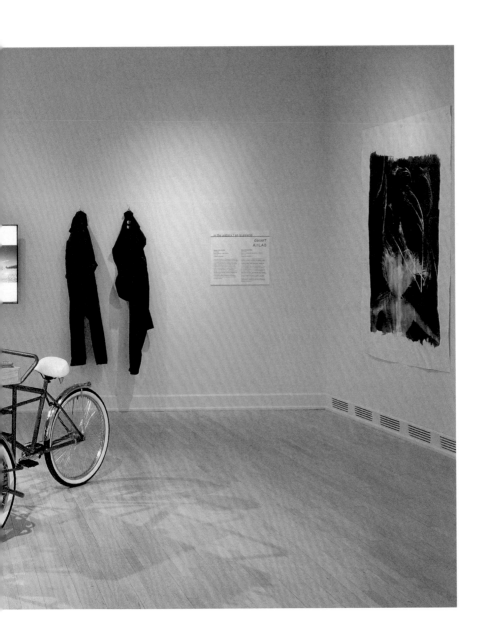

KNOWLEDGE TRANSLATOR

Further southwest, the Navajo Nation is confronting another legacy of colonial environmental exploitation: abandoned uranium mines. According to the Environmental Protection Agency, there are more than 500 abandoned uranium mines[4] on the Navajo Nation, a reservation that spans more than 27,000 square miles in Arizona, New Mexico, and Utah. Though the mines haven't been active since the 1980s, the legacy is potent. Wind exposure and runoff covers nearby communities in hazardous dust. Some homes' water supplies have elevated levels of radiation. People in these communities are at higher risk for lung and bone cancers, kidney disease, immune disorders, cardiovascular disease, and skin disorders.

Mallery Quetawki uses art to educate Indigenous peoples on these impacts. Quetawki, who is Zuni Pueblo, studied biology and art in college. When taking an anatomy course, she made large-scale, anatomically accurate pastel paintings focused on Zuni identity. After they were put on display in the Indian Health Service health center in Zuni, New Mexico, practitioners noticed something: her paintings helped their patients feel more comfortable to ask health questions. This inspired Quetawki's new career path: to use art as a bridge between Indigenous and Western knowledge to create healthier futures for Indigenous peoples.

In 2016, while working as a patient care technician at a University of New Mexico hospital, Quetawki was approached by Dr. Johnnye Lewis, director of the university's Community Environmental Health Program.[5] Dr. Lewis was working on a project to alleviate the health impacts of abandoned uranium mines on the Navajo Nation called Beesh Dootł'izh Bantsáhákees in Diné (the Navajo language), and Think Zinc in English. The goal of the multiyear research project, which is ongoing, is to measure whether supplementing zinc with people's daily diets will help mitigate the toxicity of metal exposures, particularly uranium and arsenic.

Quetawki created culturally based paintings to communicate to participants how uranium damages DNA, how zinc can repair DNA damage, and how zinc may support immune cells functions. For example, in one painting she has two strands of turquoise beads woven together, but the string is broken in the middle. The painting demonstrates that like a strand of beadwork, DNA can be mended and repaired. Too often, researchers use Indigenous communities for research but do nothing to translate and make relevant their findings to community members. This is an exploitative and patronizing model. Instead, Quetawki's art helps communicate scientific terminology or processes in a way community members can understand.

Art is not only a way to provide culturally relevant descriptions of scientific concepts; it is also useful to start conversations on stigmatized topics. "Speaking up with community members about cancer, genetics, death, and dying is very taboo," says Quetawki.

"Each tribe has a different protocol." There is a long history of outsiders exploiting tribal communities — including the uranium mining companies and past, unethical academic research — so bidirectional communication between community members and practitioners is essential to build trust.

Quetawki emphasizes, however, that her art is not just to educate Natives. It's also to educate non-Native researchers and health practitioners on the significance of Native cultures and knowledge systems. "I'm trying to inform non-Native researchers and investigators why we hold the land so sacred," said Quetawki. "We need more people with traditional knowledge to be part of the discussion when it comes to research."

IMAGINING HEALTHY FUTURES

Indigenous peoples continue to experience disproportionately high rates of chronic disease, including heart disease, asthma, diabetes, and mental health issues such as substance abuse, stress, post-traumatic stress disorder, and suicidality.[6,7] These disparities did not happen by accident. They are a direct impact of decades of intentional destruction and delegitimization of Indigenous knowledge, relationships with the land, healthcare systems, and community and political structures.

It is within this context that these artists are working to reimagine and re-create thriving, healthy communities and futures for Indigenous peoples. For Bojorquez and Quetawki, art is both a form of communication and a mode to visualize new realities.

"Instead of doing science that only bears interests to scientists, we need something of benefit to the tribe," reflects Quetawki. "We are no longer in the background, just waiting for the science. We're doing the science."

Art is one way to bring these ideas into fruition. "Art can bring a reimagination of what can be done, thinking outside of a lot of boxes or traditional disciplinary boundaries or processes," Bojorquez reflects. "Art allows us to imagine things that could never be imagined and realize those things as well."

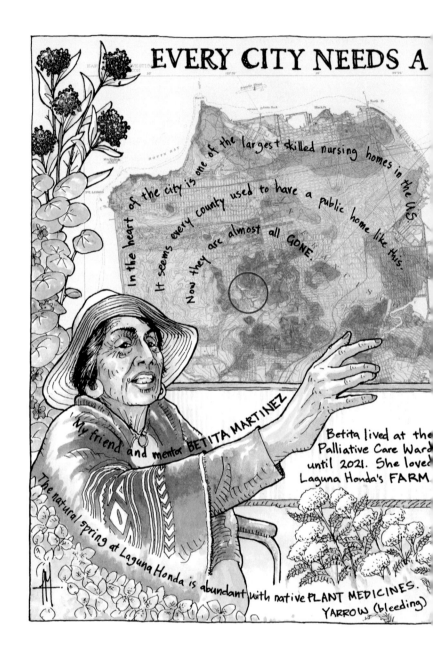

EVERY CITY NEEDS A

In the heart of the city is one of the largest skilled nursing homes in the US.

It seems every county used to have a public home like this.

Now they are almost all GONE.

My friend and mentor BETITA MARTINEZ

The natural spring at Laguna Honda is abundant with native PLANT MEDICINES.

Betita lived at the Palliative Care Ward until 2021. She loved Laguna Honda's FARM.

YARROW (bleeding)

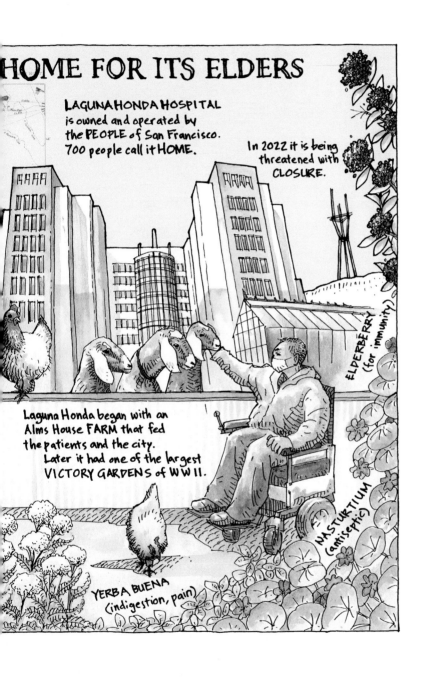

A Public Home
FERNANDO MARTÍ, M.ARCH

DREAMSPACE

When art offers a giant leap forward
for the health of all mankind.

In the *Star Trek* episode called "Miri" from 1966, Chief Medical Officer Dr. "Bones" McCoy and other members of the crew of the Starship Enterprise beam down to a 20th century Earth-like planet, nearly devoid of human life since civilization has been largely wiped out by a rogue virus. Under pressure and without access to adequate data to ensure safety, Bones manages to develop a vaccine to save the crew, many of whom have been exposed to the virus inadvertently through contact with the planet's inhabitants. It's a gripping story, even with dated special effects, and more so given our recent experiences here on Earth.

In our current day, as life imitates art due to the shared experience of COVID, this *Star Trek* episode shows the potential for making real-life science so much more engaging than textbooks ever could. Few things have been more consistently inspiring to humans this century than imagining our future in outer space.

Popular culture is replete with artistic renditions of outer space. Whether one was born during the era of *Lost in Space, Star Trek, Battlestar Galactica,* or *The Mandalorian,* we all have impressions of space in our psyche, often equated with impressions of wonder, discovery, and the future. Whenever humans are involved in that space-based future, health comes into play. In fact, space, health, and medicine are intrinsically interconnected in our minds in ways we don't even realize. Amplified and made present through the arts, the future of medicine becomes ever more tangible and relatable.

Life may imitate art, as in the example above or with *The Jetsons* foreshadowing of the age of telemedicine, but art also imitates life. The effort to grow nutritional food in deep space has been a subject of intense study on Earth and is also a key theme in the 2015 film *The Martian*, as Matt Damon's character takes a creative approach to growing vegetables in an environment inhospitable to human life.

The Translational Research Institute for Space Health (TRISH) and its team are at the very center of this Venn diagram of space, medicine, and art. TRISH is a NASA-funded organization that sponsors research, undertakes experiments, and collaborates with NASA and healthcare community innovators to plan for the quality of human health on manned missions into deep space and develop countermeasures that will prevent illness among those flying the missions to deep space. Beyond this core mission, TRISH, led by Executive Director Dorit Donoviel, Ph.D., is well aware of its importance for people here on Earth as well.

The medical advances made to support astronauts in space have a deep relevance because they portend the future of medicine for each of us as we age. In fact, all the conditions people are likely to experience as they age bear a striking resemblance to those that confront deep space astronauts. Cognitive challenges (due to a confined and isolated environment and the effect[1] of long-term space travel on brain structure and circadian rhythm), cancer (from radiation exposure), bone fragility (due to lack of gravity), nutritional deficits (due to lack of grocery shopping), loneliness and depression (due to disconnection from loved ones) are all typical concerns that astronauts face as they head out of orbit and beyond. Each of us watching NASA and other space travels on TV are likely to experience these same problems as we head into our Golden Years, albeit largely due to different factors.

TRISH is, therefore, working hand in hand with scientists, startup companies, academic innovators, and others to identify and develop preventions and cures for these issues. They test approaches on short-term space flight and analyze NASA and private astronaut data to help identify solutions to the medical hazards of space travel. In real-life space flight, there is always a physician flight surgeon aboard, although it is always possible that the physician themself will be the person who needs medical attention on what could be a three-year flight to deep space, leaving the non-medical crew to manage the crisis. If an emergency surgical intervention is required by one of the crew on the way to Mars, there is no urgent care clinic where one can stop to address a kidney stone, and there are no paramedics to call. With the recent NASA announcement[2] that astronauts on upcoming Artemis missions can be male or female and of any age between late-20s to the mid-60s, it is reasonable to assume that this cadre of space travelers will experience not just the risks of space flight, but also the travails of normal aging.

To help communicate the essential nature of their work, TRISH turned to an old-fashioned art form, film, to tell its story. In 2022, TRISH released a documentary called *Space Health: Surviving in the Final Frontier.*[3] The movie tells the story of TRISH's work through the lens of actual astronauts' personal experiences in space and how essential they feel this healthcare work is to their well-being. And, as David Hock, director of the *Space Health* documentary reminds us, "astronauts have been inhabiting the International Space Station for over 20 years. These people have lives and health issues like everyone else. Film is a medium with which most people connect and that enables the complexity of space to be explained to the non-scientific public."

Outer space is a fascinating story in and of itself. When combined with human stories, it is riveting. Added Hock: "Space is the one thing that connects the whole world. We all look at the same sky. Art, music, and culture are all part of being a healthy human, as are food and habitat. It all ties back to the story of health."

Retired astronaut Nicole Stott has a particularly keen understanding of the value of bringing space and art together to advance the experience of health. Stott had a 27-year career at NASA and participated in several space flights as well as a stint on the International Space Station (ISS) and a flight on the space shuttle before that program ended. Stott, who now serves on the TRISH Scientific Advisory Board, notably brought a small watercolor painting kit on ISS Expedition 21.

She observed that many astronauts have brought their artistic selves to space, including Cady Coleman and Ellen Ochoa, who each played flute on their missions, and Al Worden, Apollo 15 astronaut, who wrote *Hello Earth: Greetings from Endeavour*, a book that includes the poetry composed, in part, on his space journey. Alan Bean, the fourth man to set foot on the moon, became a full-time artist upon his retirement from NASA, painting pictures that were inspired by his time among the stars.

As Stott puts it, "The best problem solvers use their whole brain." She also points out that the creative arts are essential for some to ensure joy and positive mental health. On the ISS, having time to look out the window and to engage in the arts were essential for crew to stay connected and have the strength to do the work they were there to do.

Stott has literally turned her artistic interests into a healthcare mission. Initially working with the then-pediatric art director at MD Anderson Cancer Center, Ian Cion, and later through the formation of the Space for Art Foundation. Stott shared the story of sitting with an eight-year-old child at MD Anderson who, while painting, started talking about the connection between long-term space flight and her cancer experience. She related how she couldn't go outside and see friends during her long hospitalization, was subject to numerous tests, was often exposed to radiation, had very few foods she could eat, and was often separated from her family. This pointedly demonstrated to Stott "...the power of space to inspire and heal. The art itself was great, yet adding the space content really supercharged it. It allowed kids undergoing the worst possible experience to come to life and engage to talk about their illness and also their future."

A vital component of the Space for Art Foundation program is the development of space suit art, consisting of children's drawings stitched together to cover actual space suits contributed by ILC Dover LP, the maker of the garments that astronauts wear on their missions. Now there is an expanded project called "BEYOND,"[4] that includes art from children all over the world and is intended to demonstrate the connection between space, Planet Earth, climate change, and health. A recent project tied to SpaceX's Inspiration4 flight was undertaken at St. Jude Children's Research Hospital, where kids decorated an authentic space suit and now get to pass by the

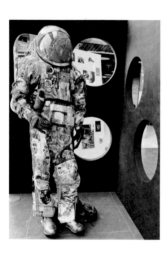

inspiring piece built by their peers as it is on permanent display in the hospital. Notably, a former St. Jude patient, Hayley Arceneaux, was a passenger on the Inspiration4 mission and is now a physician assistant at St. Jude so she can further help the kids connect to the story of space and their own futures.

Another program pioneered at St. Jude was developed in partnership with virtual reality software company Z3VR. Voices of Inspiration[5] is an immersive game, where users (aka kids with cancer) ascend to space in an elevator that takes them past walls decorated with St. Jude patient artwork. When the elevator stops, they find themselves in virtual worlds themed after questions the Inspiration4 astronauts posed to St. Jude patients before their historic launch. The idea was to help the kids feel that they were part of the mission by answering questions posed by astronauts reflective of the health challenges and fears of the children themselves, who are all cancer patients. In the game, astronaut Chris Sembroski, mission specialist, asks the kids facing their cancer treatment, and a long stay away from home, "Do you have any advice for me on dealing with nerves before a big change like this?" and the children offer their own answers back. Z3VR hopes to add biosensors to the VR headsets to surreptitiously and non-invasively measure key clinical indicators such as eye movement and heart rate, while the kids are distracted by visually amazing space scenery and gaming. Biosensors like these will also find their way into the astronauts' own gear.

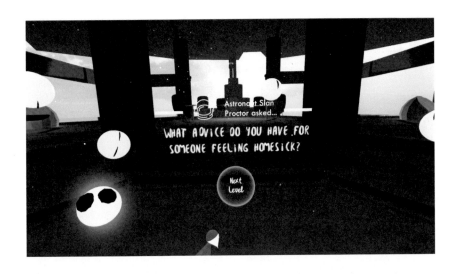

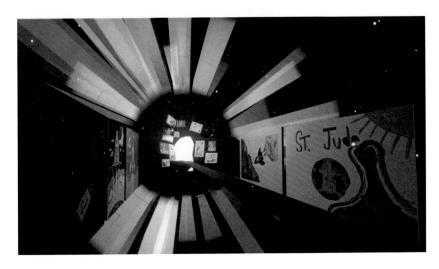

Z3VR became engaged with TRISH and the space program after a chance meeting at the South by Southwest Conference between TRISH Executive Director Donoviel and Z3VR CEO Josh Ruben. The company, which combines VR with sensors to measure medical biometrics, believes VR will be the most valuable psychiatric assessment and engagement tool ever developed. Z3VR and TRISH have focused their joint efforts on measuring eye movements, heart rate, and respiration during astronauts' exercise regimens as they prepare for their missions. The backdrop is in an immersive environment designed by artist Lucas Rizzotto, who calls himself a "creative, futurist, mad scientist." Their efforts continue with projects to measure and optimize mental health, sleep, and fitness in long-range space flight. Said Ruben: "Every virtual reality experience in the future, in fact the whole future of computing, will be based on art. It all starts with the artist's vision. Art plays a key role in public understanding and can simulate any condition, even what it's like to have a medical condition. Adding in biosensors to understand physiology increasingly adds value to the VR experience."

Notably, Z3VR is taking what they have learned from their work with astronauts and translating that into programs for the general public, the first of which is focused on sleep optimization. To reach this goal, the company has created a spin-out enterprise to develop digital therapeutics experienced through virtual reality.

TRISH has been creative about the use of art and culture to expand awareness of the importance of its work. Among the best examples is the art created out of the Inspiration4 astronauts' medical data by renowned digital artist Refik Anadol, who uses data as a medium. The series of works, called *An Important Memory for Humanity,*[6] is a non-fungible token (NFT) art collection that turned the space biomedical research data into gorgeous artistic renderings.

"In my art practice, I collaborate with machine intelligence to construct new ways of perceiving our environments that might eventually enhance our collective well-being," explained Anadol. "*An Important Memory for Humanity* gave me a chance to take this goal to a new level by both revealing an insight into the challenges of space travel for the human body and contributing to a meaningful cause to help solve some health issues on Earth. It was such an honor to visualize the cutting-edge research conducted by TRISH on the impact that the conditions in space had on the astronauts and create meaningful NFTs that enabled us to donate to St. Jude Children's Research Hospital."

The NFT project was the brainchild of James Hury III, Ph.D., deputy director of TRISH. Hury knew there would be a great deal of biomedical research data captured on the Inspiration4 flight. While it would be used to advance medical research for future missions, Hury felt it important to elevate the data in a way that made it more approachable and meaningful.

By delivering the biomedical data in an artistic form, the team could turn mundane data into interesting and relatable concepts that amplify awareness to, and in appreciation of, the scientific advancements necessary to ensure the safety of future long-range space flight. Additionally, since space travel offers a testing ground for medical advances that apply on Earth, Hury thought it could be possible to use artistic renderings of the data to show the physical effects of space on longevity and make it more meaningful to the broader Earth-bound audience.

Hury connected with J. Harry Edmiston, an award-winning creative director, producer, and photographer, who engaged artist Anadol. During the Inspiration4 flight, as with all current space travel, medical experiments were conducted on the crew, in this case using hand-held ultrasound devices from Butterfly Network, Inc. and biometrics collected via Apple Watch. The result was a series of unique artistic works intended to interpret the health data from Inspiration4's crew in a uniquely accessible way to show the physical effect of space travel. One NFT image features side-by-side aspects of all four astronauts' ultrasound scans, visually highlighting their similarities and differences. Another combines the crew's collective biometric data into a sweeping collage that never stops moving. These artistic renderings give an unusual and beautiful perspective of the impact of space on health, amplifying the essential nature of the efforts to advance research to

care for astronauts, but also humans in general. Notes Edmiston: "In the field of medicine, the data is so rich. So it makes a lot of sense to use it to raise attention to this area of research. This project is as much about instigating creativity and change as it is about the actual work."

Notably, Anadol's stunning images were auctioned after the Inspiration4 voyage and raised millions of dollars for St. Jude and to fund further TRISH medical research.

Dylan Mathis, communication manager for NASA's International Space Station Program, comments that art, and especially immersive art experiences, "...conveys the awe and wonder of space at such a visceral level." What lies beyond our atmosphere inspires a level of creativity and imagination that can actively change health outcomes when applied to the field.

Programs such as those of TRISH and the Space Art Foundation, as well as the efforts of the many collaborators with whom they have worked, demonstrate how important art can be to telling the story of the humans involved in space flight. And where there are humans, there is a need for attention to their health and welfare. The intersection of art, science, medicine, and outer space is a natural one. As it draws our eyes and explorations skyward, it also expands our ambitions, our accomplishments, and our sense of wonder about what it is possible to achieve in this lifetime and on our own planet.

8.0

ACTION

PAPERWEIGHT

"The vehicle is art, the public act is activism
and the debt alleviation is direct action."

— MSCHF Chief Creative Officer Kevin Wiesner

In the early days of the pandemic when vaccines were still a distant possibility and hospitals were newly overflowing with seriously ill and dying people, the avant-garde art collective MSCHF (pronounced "mischief") dropped its first digital zine, *Volume 1: Bread*. In between guides to creating universal basic income by scamming Spotify and how to drive a hearse for Uber to maximize profits by not following traffic laws, MSCHF solicited readers who owed more than $50,000 in medical debt to send in their bills to the creators. The appeal for medical debtors was styled in the form of a medical bill, with "final notice" marked at the bottom of the page.

Of all the challenges with the U.S. healthcare system, the financial burden is arguably the most troubling. The U.S. has the most expensive healthcare system in the world for public and commercial insurers — and also for patients. The U.S. spends roughly double per person on healthcare than other wealthy countries. Medical bills loom large in the psyche of Americans — both as physical documents, embodied in stacks of multicolored, threatening notices, and as the failure of health insurance to truly protect us from financial risk. Euphemistically titled "Explanation of Benefits" letters arrive in the mail from health insurers, announcing the end of a byzantine process designed to eke out the maximum profit and minimum benefits possible, with patients at the end of a long chain of abdicated responsibility. These EOBs are followed by bills and all too often referrals to collections, bad credit, and bankruptcies. For the uninsured, the bills come directly from their healthcare providers.

The sheer volume of paper generated by this process lends itself to art. Artists and activists have been activated by the visual and visceral nature of medical bills, debts, and unjust practices that leave patients holding the bag in an unaffordable system, leading to financial distress and ever-worsening health outcomes. The nonprofit organization Americans for the Arts notes that artists and other creative professionals are themselves more likely to be part of the 40% of Americans who are uninsured or underinsured.

Six months after their call for submissions MSCHF dropped its next project: *Three Medical Bills*. Commissioned as large-scale oil paintings, the artworks included each line item of the bills, ranging from blood draws to various enigmatic discounts, and were made available in a virtual gallery online called Medical Bill Art. "The process of making art in the gallery ecosystem is the process of creating value. By making a bill into a painting, MSCHF set two monetary forces equal and opposite one another, thereby nullifying the bill," explained the artists.

The sale itself continued the exhibition: Otis, a distributed art ownership platform, purchased *Three Medical Bills* and offered crowdfunded, shared ownership of the artwork at $20 per share. By the end of 2020, 3,750 shares had been sold,[1] and the offering was closed. In total, MSCHF raised $73,360.36 to pay off the medical bills of three people, by "transforming the lines, numbers, and words of the bill into oil paint on canvas." For now, neither MSCHF nor Otis plans to repeat the process with any additional medical bills. While just three people had medical debt wiped out in this installation, the virality-by-design of the project resulted in greater awareness of the ever-growing problem of medical debt in the U.S., which MSCHF describes as "both a bill and a painting are currency in a vast, complex system for the movement of wealth."

The zine's project helped to expose the absurdity of the medical billing and medical debt that burdens 100 million people in the U.S., or every four in 10 adults, as reported by the Kaiser Family Foundation,[2] and refocus attention on a problem that many have become desensitized to after years of headlines. Medical debt is hard to measure because it shows up on credit card bills as well as in overdue billing notices and debt sold off to collection agencies, yet it is estimated that almost $200 billion is currently owed by Americans. Unsurprisingly, the debt burden is not equitably distributed — women, Black, and Latino Americans hold most of the medical debt. Uninsured people are more likely to have medical debt than insured people, but health insurance does not fully protect people from debt.

In 2022, the three major credit reporting bureaus announced that they would change the way medical debts in collections are reported and show up in credit scores starting in 2023, giving consumers a small leg up when it comes to negotiating overdue debts and mitigating the impact on their other finances. Unfortunately these changes do little to tackle the burden and negative consequences of medical debt on Americans, which continues to account for more than half of all bankruptcy filings.[3]

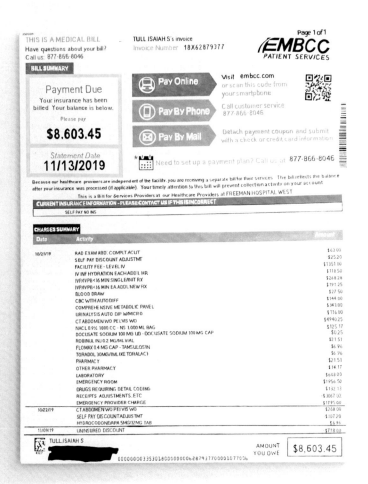

THIS IS A MEDICAL BILL
Have questions about your bill?
Call us: 877-866-8046

TULL ISAIAH S's invoice
Invoice Number 18X62879377

Page 1 of 1

EMBCC
PATIENT SERVICES

BILL SUMMARY

Payment Due
Your insurance has been billed. Your balance is below.
Please pay

$8,603.45

Statement Date
11/13/2019

Pay Online — Visit embcc.com or scan this code from your smartphone

Pay By Phone — Call customer service 877-866-8046

Pay By Mail — Detach payment coupon and submit with a check or credit card information

Need to set up a payment plan? Call us at 877-866-8046

Because our healthcare providers are independent of the facility, you are receiving a separate bill for their services. The bill reflects the balance after your insurance was processed (if applicable). Your timely attention to this bill will prevent collection activity on your account.

This is a Bill for Services Providers at our Healthcare Providers at FREEMAN HOSPITAL WEST

CURRENT INSURANCE INFORMATION - PLEASE CONTACT US IF THIS IS INCORRECT

SELF PAY NO INS

CHARGES SUMMARY

Date	Activity	Amount
10/21/19	RAD EXAM ABD: COMPLT ACUT	$63.00
	SELF PAY DISCOUNT ADJUSTMT	-$25.20
	FACILITY FEE - LEVEL IV	$1351.00
	IV INF HYDRATION EACH ADD'L HR	$118.50
	IVP/IVPB <16 MIN SINGLE/INIT RX	$268.28
	IVP/IVPB <16 MIN EA ADDL NEW RX	$191.25
	BLOOD DRAW	$27.50
	CBC WITH AUTO DIFF	$144.00
	COMPREHENSIVE METABOLIC PANEL	$343.00
	URINALYSIS AUTO DIP W/MICRO	$116.00
	CT ABDOMEN WO PELVIS WO	$4940.25
	NACL 0.9% 1000 CC - NS 1,000 ML BAG	$125.17
	DOCUSATE SODIUM 100 MG UD - DOCUSATE SODIUM 100 MG CAP	$0.25
	ROBINUL INJ 0.2 MG/ML VIAL	$21.51
	FLOMAX 0.4 MG CAP - TAMSULOSIN	$6.96
	TORADOL 30MG/1ML (XE TORALAC)	$6.96
	PHARMACY	$21.51
	OTHER PHARMACY	$14.17
	LABORATORY	$603.00
	EMERGENCY ROOM	$1956.50
	DRUGS REQUIRING DETAIL CODING	$132.13
	RECEIPTS ADJUSTMENTS ,ETC	-$3067.02
	EMERGENCY PROVIDER CHARGE	$1795.00
10/22/19	CT ABDOMEN WO PELVIS WO	$268.00
	SELF PAY DISCOUNT ADJUSTMT	$107.20
	HYDROCODONE/APA 5MG/32MG TAB	$6.96
11/09/19	UNINSURED DISCOUNT	$718.00

TULL,ISAIAH S

AMOUNT YOU OWE **$8,603.45**

00000000335301800000000628743770000107705

MEDICAL DEBT AND THE COST OF CARE: "IT'S STILL THE PRICES, STUPID."

The heavy burden of medical debt is directly related to the skyrocketing cost of healthcare in the U.S., and high prices are the main reason why the U.S. spends more on healthcare than any other country.

The U.S. now spends more than $4 trillion on healthcare per year. The late Uwe Reinhardt, Ph.D., and collaborators published a seminal analysis of health-care spending, availability of resources, and utilization in 2003 called "It's The Prices, Stupid." After his death, his co-authors updated the data in 2019,[4] reconfirming the findings and showing the ever-growing divide between the U.S. and other countries. Fundamentally, the prices for the same or comparable doctor's visits, hospital stays, procedures and surgeries, medical technology, and pharmaceuticals are simply higher in the U.S. than in other countries; they are often exponentially more expensive. Furthermore, those much higher prices result in worse health out-comes in domains ranging from excess mortality, affordability, equity, access, and quality of care, according to The Commonwealth Fund.

Our unaffordable healthcare system hurts patients — so much so that the term "financial toxicity" has been used to describe the financial burden and distress of the high cost of treatment on patients seeking care. Financial toxicity shows up in anxiety, stress, and depression; skipping or rationing critical medications or care; food inse-curity; and, of course, medical debt.

The complex causes and effects of our unaffordable healthcare system are as abstract and distant as a policy debate, yet the impact is clear for Americans. Financial toxicity shows up in everyday lives as the high cost of care, medical bills, and debt. Activists and people engaging in mutual aid (community self-support efforts) have been addressing the downstream issues that show up in Americans' lives — paying for unexpected care needs by sharing GoFundMe posts, or directly helping pay off medical debts. GoFundMe reports that a third of all fundraisers are related to medical bills,[5] but most fundraisers don't net much money. Furthermore, the GoFundMe campaigns that go viral and net up-wards of millions of dollars combine the tools of marketing, compelling visual elements, and expert storytelling to get strangers interested. And, as report-ed in the American Journal of Public Health,[6] campaigns in 2020 raised substantially less money in areas with greater medical debt, higher uninsur-ance rates, and lower incomes.

TELLING STORIES OF MEDICAL DEBT AND DEBT FORGIVENESS

Jared Walker stitched a response[7] in early 2021 to the popular TikTok prompt, "What's a piece of information you learned that feels illegal to know?" In less than a minute, he explained that nonprofit hospitals must have a charity care policy that forgives medical bills for people with very low incomes and quickly showed followers how to apply for these financial assistance programs. Walker's one-minute TikTok reached more than 30 million people and brought visibility to his organization, Dollar For. This nonprofit group has created a user-friendly system for medical bill self-help as well as a volunteer-supported medical bill negotiation lab[8] built around the charity care policies mandated by the Affordable Care Act and an understanding of the slippery tactics consumer debt collectors follow when reaching out to patients.

Dollar For has been featured multiple times on the podcast *An Arm and a Leg,* the show about why healthcare costs "so freaking much, and what we can (maybe) do about it," led by veteran public broadcasting journalist Dan Weissmann and supported by the nonprofit Kaiser Health News. In nearly 100 episodes to date, *An Arm and a Leg* breaks down the intentionally opaque and tangled issues around the cost of care in compelling stories and plain language while providing action-oriented steps that patients can take to avoid unnecessary bills in spite of a harmful system. Weissmann speaks to advocates on the show like Laurie Todd, who calls herself The Insurance Warrior and helps people get their insurance companies to pay for treatment based on enforcing the complex terms of their agreements, filing appeals, and finding past precedent for treatments being covered. Recently, they launched First Aid Kit, a newsletter that distills down the learnings from the show's guests to help people fight the high cost of healthcare in their own lives. On the power of storytelling

about healthcare costs, Weissmann says, "It's the most ginormous story — it affects just about everybody, in the most intimate and dramatic ways. It's both a really, really human story, and a really, really big-picture story."

SUBVERTING THE SYSTEM: ACTIVISM, MUTUAL AID, AND ART

Jerry Ashton had spent four decades in the credit and collections industry when he encountered the Occupy Wall Street crowds in Manhattan's Zuccotti Park in 2011 and learned about activists' plans for mutual aid to pay off medical debts. This inspired Ashton and a colleague, Craig Antico, to find a way to abolish the burden of medical debts entirely. While Dollar For's solution tackles debt forgiveness at the hospital or provider level for patients, RIP Medical Debt goes even further downstream by purchasing bulk medical debt in the millions from hospitals and collections agencies at pennies on the dollar and forgiving debts entirely. Through this arbitrage model, they say that a $100 donation forgives $10,000 in medical debt, using the toxic medical debt system against itself.

In 2018, the comedian John Oliver featured RIP Medical Debt on his show, *Last Week Tonight,* about predatory medical debt acquisition and collections. In the show, which typically uses satire, exposition, and unexpected visual elements to address complex social and political topics, Oliver partnered with RIP Medical Debt to create a debt acquisition company and forgive $15 million in medical debt for 9,000 people. In the episode, Oliver explained how he took advantage of the lack of regulations around debt acquisition in many states to start a company he called Central Asset Recovery Professionals, Inc., or "CARP, after the bottom-feeding fish," in order to buy the medical debt, which was out-of-statute, meaning that the debtors could no longer be sued for the uncollected debts, even though companies like CARP could still buy and attempt to collect on the debt. At the end of the episode, in a grandiose ceremony reminiscent of classic TV game shows like *The Price is Right*, Oliver forgives the debt surrounded by spinning gold dollar signs and bills falling from the sky. To date, the episode has more than 17 million views on YouTube in addition to the millions of views through HBO's cable and digital channels.

As of August 2022, RIP Medical Debt reports forgiving $6.7 billion in medical debts.[9] In a surreal turn, hospitals are beginning to donate medical debt directly to the organization to achieve debt forgiveness and reduce financial toxicity for patients. While RIP Medical Debt's approach doesn't prevent the causes of medical debt, it is alleviating the most persistent and harmful debts when all other approaches have failed.

The conceptual artist Cassie Thornton was also inspired by an Occupy Wall Street debt resistance group, Strike Debt (now known as the Debt Collective), to examine the relationship between financial debt and unconscious thoughts. Thornton developed mental models of how debt is visualized by debtors and created objects and architectural installations like piñatas and soundscapes to help people understand that debt is a political subject, not just a personal issue. Her latest project, The Hologram, imagines a new model for delivering healthcare in a post-capitalist, peer-to-peer system that honors the physical, mental, and social health of people and treats caring for people's health as therapeutic and financially valuable itself. Visually, The Hologram is a three-dimensional triangle, meant to represent three people who meet on a regular basis, to listen to and support the physical, mental, and social health of the fourth person, who is "The Hologram." Thornton's work and the "social technology" of The Hologram reinforces the role that artists play in experimenting with revolutionary new ideas and social change.

The ephemera of medical bills and the more enduring plague of medical debt obscures the deeper question: What is healthcare worth, and who deserves to access it? One community grappling with these questions, The O+ (O Positive) Festival was founded near the Catskills, New York, in 2010 by a small group of artists-activists, doctors, and a dentist to exchange "the art of medicine for the medicine of art" and has since grown into a national nonprofit organization dedicated to helping un- and underinsured artists and creatives exchange art and performance for healthcare services. Their community-centered work seeks to help neighbors take control of their collective well-being through the exchange of art, music, and wellness, and each festival includes a large public health fair and other activities designed to promote well-being. The O+ approach reminds us that the pursuit of individual and community health goes far beyond the hospital doors and decenters the role of money, medical bills, and debt in providing healthcare to our neighbors and communities.

Recent changes to laws and regulations like the No Surprises Act and to the credit reporting system will protect patients from a portion of unexpected and unjust medical bills. However, the problem of medical debt remains tightly intertwined with America's overpriced healthcare system and a culture of medicine and healthcare delivery that ignores the harm of financial toxicity on patients.

To address the worst inequities in our healthcare system, art, creative expression, and activism offer a measure of hope and opportunity for change.

I see my own mother, Judi Bari, in this throughline of art and activism. She was a self-taught graphic designer who used her ability to quickly create eye-catching flyers and signs for anti-war protests and community organizing meetings. Later in her life, she turned the protest music of the earlier 20th century labor union movement into songs about stopping clearcutting of ancient redwood forests and demanding that the FBI and the Oakland Police investigate the attack on her life that almost killed her, all while leading the environmental movement in Northern California to monumental success in protecting Headwaters Forest. Art and activism were entwined in our lives.

Tragically, my mother died of cancer before her activism could evolve to meet the pressing challenges of today.

My mother spent her life calling attention to the deep imbalances of money and power, first as a union organizer and then as the protector of Northern California's quickly disappearing redwood forests. Like many activists, she used the tools of art and music to capture the public's attention and make complex and difficult topics urgent and accessible. Similarly, today's artists and activists tackling medical debt and the cost of healthcare are working to break through the noise and push back on a cruel and unaffordable system that must be countered through creative expression and collective action.

We need artists to help us imagine a more humane, equitable healthcare future and activists to accelerate this change. Artists and activists are changemakers in our society; they are truth-tellers using many forms of expression.

ON WHAT IS POSSIBLE

From a conversation with Emily F. Peters,
edited for clarity.

Incrementalism versus radical change is what I'm thinking about right now.

Incrementalism feels most comfortable, especially in medicine. The ability to make radical change is very hard for us. The way that it has been built, this apprenticeship model, this hierarchical model.

Medicine is very boundaried. We often think about things in ways that we've thought about them before. Our solutions tend to be incremental solutions because we're moving bit by bit on a pathway that's predestined, that we know.

If we want to change the ways we deliver care or address the needs of certain populations or dismantle the hierarchies that we see, we need to be much more radical. What we're lacking from a little bit is the idea of what is possible.

Part of changing others' mindsets is getting people out of the common medical world that they work with into a different kind of realm. One of the benefits from my practice transformation work at Mount Sinai Health System is that I had a multidisciplinary team. I worked with designers, engineers, data analysts — not just our usual teams of nurses and doctors.

Part of the reason we had some success is because they would ask provocative questions that would shift the way that we thought. The solution for radical change in medicine requires us to bring in people from different fields.

Why isn't there an artist on a practice transformation and improvement team? They would push us to think about something and think about it in a different way. One of the things art does well is it thinks outside the boundaries.

If you really want to change healthcare, you have to do it from the outside in. And yet healthcare is incredibly resistant to outside-in change.

I feel like an "insider outsider" to healthcare personally. It's part of why I will always make sure I'm able to keep seeing patients, to keep that perspective. One group that's well poised to do an outside-in change in healthcare is patients. Patients are the secret link in all of this. And it just so happens we're all patients.

Ultimately, no one's coming to save us in healthcare. We have to save ourselves. There's a real desire that I have to pour into our communities and to pour into people who are doing this work in a real, sustainable way.

We have so much to fix. For example, insulin costs more now than it ever did before, and people are dying from an inability to get insulin. People are now fighting getting vaccines when vaccines have literally changed the course of public health for hundreds of years. We're going backwards. We've made all these wonderful discoveries, and yet we're going backwards. We can't leave the next generation with these problems when they'll also have the problems of world wars and climate change.

If nothing else, I want us to have pushed far enough forward in terms of improving equity in healthcare, where you could look at your kid and say, "I did my best."

I hope we work hard to do our collective best.

Looking Ahead
JAMES LEE CHIAHAN

Protein structures and user interface elements in this artwork are inspired by Foldit, a revolutionary crowdsourcing computer game[1] enabling the general public to contribute to ongoing medical research. Scientists use results from the game to treat diseases and advance innovations, proving that the future of medicine is participatory.

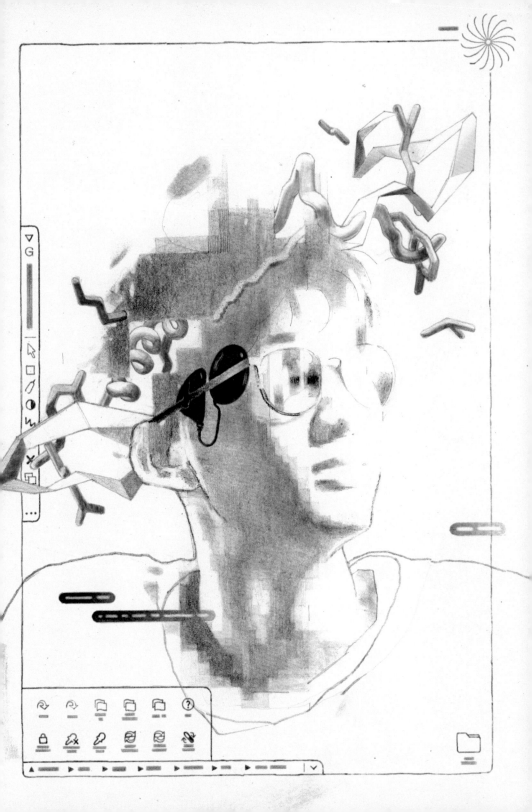

INSIDE JOB

Practicing the art of change within healthcare systems.

All of us who are part of healthcare, whether patients with lived experience, frontline nurses, doctors, policy makers, or executives, have the capacity to be change leaders.

For all of my career, I've focused on facilitating change within healthcare. While the titles have varied (head of innovation, executive director of engage-ment, etc.), the core theme has been to bring about change. These roles and projects start with the excitement and behest of a leader who sees an opportunity to do new things, fix old things, or a combination of the two. I've been a part of work that has brought me deep, rewarding joy and work that has been some of the more painful moments of my professional life.

Innovation, like art, is subjective. It can be simple or complex. It can make us feel a range of emotions, including joy, comfort, discomfort, and even pain. Sometimes we seek it out, and sometimes we find it — even when we aren't looking for it.

Facilitating change — particularly in the risk-adverse world of healthcare — has felt like a form of art. That isn't to say everything I've been a part of has been beautiful or melodious. Like art, innovation can be difficult to create and hard to experience.

To explore the connection between change and art more deeply, I sat down with two friends, colleagues and collaborators for this story — both of them leaders of change in healthcare. First, I spoke with Susannah Fox who led innovation at the U.S. Department of Health and Human Services in the federal government. Fox has been on the cutting edge of the patient empowerment movement since its earliest days. She speaks candidly, yet also with wit and humor, about her experiences helping every part of healthcare more deeply value the lived experiences of people affected by disease, trauma, and frontline care.

I also spoke with Adam Dole, who has spearheaded several healthcare startups and nonprofits. Dole has always modeled a heart-based style of leadership and vision. As a Presidential Innovation Fellow under President Obama, he helped champion the creation of Blue Button, a standard that lets patients download their own medical records. Today at Bento he is leading an organization focused on what he calls "an absurd problem," food insecurity in the richest nation in the world.

What follows are insights from the conversation I had with both Fox and Dole about their own experiences, along with my own reflections on leading change. There are also three exercises for you, designed to be explored in the order in which they are presented, to help you channel your inner artist as a champion of change in your own world.

PRACTICE MAKES BETTER

Early in our discussion of art, change, and healthcare, Fox smartly pointed out that both artists and clinicians use the word *practice* to describe their work. She added that BJ Miller, a renowned palliative care physician, talks about palliative care as an explicitly creative practice, saying, "My purpose is to reach out across disciplines and invite design thinking into this big conversation. That is, to bring intention and creativity to the experience of dying."[1] Dole spoke about teamwork as being like a dance and pointed out that communication between a doctor and patient is, in a way, a form of art, almost a live improv act. Designers also talk about their work as a *practice,* something that is easy to learn, yet mastery comes from a lifetime of experience.

My own training and experience is rooted in the practice of human-centered design. In this field, we focus on putting people most affected by a problem or opportunity at the center of solving or creating. The exercises here are drawn from some of the same tools we use in this design process.

How do you ease into this kind of human-centered healthcare design practice? Any good coach or teacher will agree that practicing something new is best when we feel safe and the stakes are low. Musicians often practice in solo, sound-isolated practice rooms, while artists might doodle in a sketchbook before putting their brush to the canvas. Practicing something new when you are emotionally invested (i.e., the stakes are high as with nearly everything in healthcare) is a challenge.

One team I led, which was charged with teaching every staff member the basics of human-centered design, always started with having students reimagine the employee badge. No one had any strong sense of owner-ship or investment in the badge, but it is something everyone wore every day and, as a result, had feelings about how it could be improved. It was a safe place to start practicing.

When it came time to teach brain-storming, we began with the basics of improv theater. Always saying "yes, and...", the practice of improv, like dance, is about supporting your partner and accepting the premise of whatever wild statement comes out of their mouth. That agreement of safety makes it easier to come up with new, bold, and creative ideas.

As you approach the concepts and exercises in this chapter, try to think of them as a form of low-stakes prac-tice. Think of them as a first improv lesson, the first dance steps, or the first time picking up a musical instru-ment. Give yourself permission to be a little messy, wonderfully imperfect, and relentlessly curious.

A CONVERSATION BETWEEN OUR HEART AND HEAD

When I led innovation at the Johns Hopkins Sibley Innovation Hub, we had a standard practice for new members of our team. We sent them to one of the hospital floors with a blank note-book and asked them to sit somewhere out of the way and sketch whatever they saw over the course of a few hours. Almost always, they came back with powerful observations and a list of questions. They had gained a curiosity and perspective on what they'd seen.

Fox, an early leader in the patient-centered care movement, told me art is tied to this practice of gaining perspective. "It is a daily critical ques-tion," looking at something which has to be explored and examined. "Art is a practice of curiosity ... a way of seeing. [Making art] is how we learn things."

Facilitating change starts the same way. We learn to change our perspec-tive, to see the world differently. That perspective shift can come from gaining empathy — the practice of seeking to understand the world as someone else experiences it. It can also come from simply being present and observing. In the world of healthcare, having a *critical question* starts simply with an interest in how someone else is expe-riencing something. How does a nurse feel about his shift or a new proto-col? How does a patient feel about the news a doctor just delivered? How does someone without access to essentials, like safe housing or food, feel about navigating their daily life? Asking curious *critical questions* about the lives and experiences of others is crucial to understanding how change will affect them.

I once led a project aimed at under-standing and addressing the health needs of people living in Washington, D.C.'s most economically challenged neighborhoods. We asked members of the community things like "How do you define health and well-being?" and "What are your barriers to living your best days?" What we heard were impactful, often heart-touching stories of challenges in daily life, which were way more fundamental than getting to a doctor. When we shared those stories and insights with our healthcare colleagues and leaders, they sat up. We had their attention. The stories made it a lot easier to ask for funding for new programs aimed at empowering members of the community to solve for those fundamental needs. Without that process, it is likely the health system would have simply built new doctors' offices in the neighborhood — an investment which would have been a waste to both the community and health system.

When I first hired an artist in residence, we had to navigate a new employment model. As a musician, she was used to creating on her own and being paid to perform her creations. As an organization, we were used to hiring employees and contractors for a job or scope of work, which the employer would ultimately own. We had to craft a new type of agreement that allowed her to continue to explore and own her artistic mission while being paid to be part of our team's work. Her different perspective created change in our organization from the very start, as we had to develop more innovative contracts to even begin collaborating.

As change leaders, we have to use both our hearts and our heads. We have to borrow the artist's practice of gaining curiosity and perspective. We use what we find to create something that triggers an emotional response in our audience. And then we connect those emotions to clear calls to concise actions. Impactful change comes when we connect the emotions

shared about something we observe to the actions we want to inspire.

EXERCISE: HEART AND HEAD

The opposite page contains a Heart and Head exercise. Use the space provided in this book to begin to explore a part of your healthcare world and create a call to action.

1. Begin by completing the sentence: Today, I am curious about...
2. Go to a place where you can explore that curiosity (a waiting room, a nursing floor, a treatment area, an office space, a place where you care for someone else, a research lab, etc.). Sit quietly and begin to observe. What do you see? What do you hear? What do you feel?
3. Capture your observations. It could be a simple sketch, a list of sounds, or a reflection of feelings. Channel your inner child.
4. After some time (maybe a few minutes or even a day), address the remaining prompts.

OUR WORK AND MISSION

The act of creating something, particularly something driven by an emotional inspiration, can be exhilarating. As Dole describes it, "When I put something into the world and see it take root and grow it brings me joy." He said it is what keeps him optimistic and moving forward. Fox describes herself as an *impact junkie* — someone who is most excited when she's helping transform healthcare into something more human.

TODAY, I AM CURIOUS ABOUT...

While sitting quietly and observing, what do you see? What do you hear? What do you feel? Use this space below to capture those observations as a drawing, mind map, song lyrics... anything!

1. WHAT I OBSERVED MADE ME FEEL:

2. THAT FEELING MATTERS BECAUSE:

3. WHAT I WOULD LIKE TO SEE CHANGED IS:

4. THAT CHANGE WILL HAVE A POSITIVE IMPACT BECAUSE:

For most change leaders I know, regardless of their confidence translating new ideas into actions in the world can feel like they're an artist debuting their latest work. Their ideas become subject to praise, questioning, critique, and ridicule. Often what they create challenges existing views, mental models, and norms. For a lot of change leaders and artists, gaining awareness of their complex cycle of feelings is the key to a long career and greater impact.

"When [people tell us no, they won't support us] it tests my optimism. We're in the world for too short of a time to not try to do this." That's how Dole put it when speaking about his calls to action being rejected. I remember having a conversation with one of our artists after a big presentation of our work where they said, "These things just take it out of me, I need a few days to recuperate before I can really be productive again." I understood exactly what they meant. The work leading up to the presentation included hearing powerfully emotional stories from patients and caregivers who had experienced pain and suffering. We had to not only honor those stories, but also use them as a call for action. It was an uncomfortable presentation because it meant holding up a mirror to some of our organization's own processes and leaders.

"Pain with a purpose is what change looks like," Fox said when we spoke about the challenges of trying to lead change when an audience might be resistant to the work. Artists and innovators shouldn't shy away from painful emotions involved in the practice, but they also can't rely on the emotions being the only case for change.

"Emotions are necessary, but not sufficient. They create an initial appeal to a challenge, but they aren't always what drives action," said Dole. "I have to also make the problem matter to a CFO in a way that can't be brushed away." He wants emotion to translate into action.

Fox brought up Sorrel King, whose daughter, Josie, died of a preventable mistake in a hospital. When King speaks to groups, she starts by declaring, "I'm not here to make you cry, I'm here to make you take action." She knows her daughter's story is emotionally powerful. She knows it will tug at the heartstrings of her audience. But she wants to use that emotional pull to drive change.

Most people working in healthcare aren't tasked with innovation, change, or strategy. But all of us are capable of holding a vision for how we want to see care improved. For instance, your *work* may be nursing, but you can also have a *mission* for the change you want to see. That mission may not be directly part of your work; however, it can still help sustain your optimism and progress to continue practicing change.

ART AND CHANGE CAN
BE SNEAKY

Leading change in healthcare presents unique challenges. Often we feel constrained by our role or position in an organization. Sometimes we encounter resistance, which can be appropriate when dealing with people's lives and well-being. Effective change leaders and artists become adept at working within constraints.

Once, a frontline nurse approached our team hoping for a solution to preventable IV line infections. When prompted for her own ideas, she told us more nurses needed to remember to wipe the injection ports on the lines with disinfectant before inserting a needle. She thought a fun drawing might help. We encouraged her to take a stab at creating something, and she produced a wonderful cartoonish IV hub doing the twist with a caption that read, "Remember to scrub the hub."

The best part about the *Do the Twist* drawing was its simplicity. It was hand-drawn art that could be copied on a copier at the nurses station. She began making copies and posting them anywhere there were IV lines in patients' arms. It was a hit, and it worked.

"Artists find a way to be sneaky," says Fox. She says the same is true of people leading change. Sometimes, we have to find a way to slip our call to action into our everyday work.

Fox also referenced Andrew Simonet, author of *Making Your Life as an Artist* and founder of Artists U, a collaborative focused on helping artists make both an impact and a sustainable living. Simonet said, "Your mission as an artist is what you're trying to give to the world — a way of moving, hearing, seeing, and collaborating. Without clarity about this mission in your work, you cannot tap into your most authentic self. That understanding of what drives you helps sustain your artistic life and career over the long haul."[2]

EXERCISE: YOUR MISSION
FOR CHANGE

On the following page there is a Mission activity. The goal is to help you identify your mission as a change leader and to see how the work you do in your professional career may be a means toward accomplishing that mission.

1. Read the prompts, but before filling them out, take a moment for a mindful activity. Take a walk, sit quietly, or listen to peaceful music. Do something that gives you a moment to think.
2. Fill out the prompts honestly. These are for you and you alone. Try to avoid self-censoring or being self-critical.
3. Try to avoid boiling the ocean; focus on the simple.
4. Optional: remove this page and keep it somewhere.

TO ME, HEALTHCARE MEANS...

....

SOME OF MY MOST STRONGLY HELD VALUES INCLUDE:

....

....

....

I BELIEVE .... WILL BE IMPROVED WHEN:

....

BECAUSE:

....

MY HEALTHCARE MISSION IS TO CHANGE:

....

FOR:

....

SO THAT:

....

EXERCISE: BE A LITTLE SNEAKY

In the first exercise, you borrowed from artists the ability to be intentionally curious about some part of your world. In the second, you developed your mission for change. Now, it is time to create some art.

Use a blank piece of paper to create something based on the first two exercises. The catch? Once you've created your art, see if you can sneak it in somewhere special, with the hope that someone will find it and feel inspired. If you post it on social media, tag @procedurepress, and we'll help share it.

Your art can be anything you like. It can be a poem, a song, a drawing, origami, or something entirely of your own creation. Maybe you were inspired by what you saw in a doctor's office waiting room, and you have an idea for changing something in the lives of the people waiting. What might you make and slip into a stack of magazines?

1. Reflect on what you observed in exercise #1 (Heart and Head). What did you see and hear and feel? What emotions did you observe? How did you frame those observations and emotions as a case for change?
2. Reflect on your own personal mission for change from exercise #2. What do you want to change in the world as a result of what you observed and felt?
3. Now, create something, anything, for someone else to experience. Maybe you want them to feel the same emotions you felt and share your mission for change. Maybe you want to inspire them to take action.
4. Take a photo of the page, now your work of art, and share it somewhere you hope someone will find it.

Leading change in healthcare, much like creating art, is an emotional, creative, mission-driven process. It can happen anywhere and come from anyone — from patients with their own lived experience to senior leaders.

By borrowing from the same tools and mindsets used by artists, we can create powerful, mission-based calls to action and rewarding impact. Sometimes that change means doing something new, sometimes it means doing something in a different way, and sometimes it is about fixing or modernizing something old. Just like art, sometimes the change we make can be simple, affecting only our own work or life. And sometimes it can be grand in scale.

In my experience, facilitating change — particularly in the risk-adverse world of healthcare — has felt like a form of art. Like art, change can be difficult to create and hard to experience, not always beautiful or melodious. I hope that the stories and exercises here inspire you to find new ways to practice innovation, to shift perspectives, to find power in what can sometimes be painful, and to be creative in how to make change happen.

Epilogue
EMILY F. PETERS

It is quite the cliché that the conclusion of a book reveals the characters were connected all along. Art and medicine, together, entangled throughout time.

This wasn't what I set out to write at the start. This was to be a book about endurance. How to "stay in the game" — how to practice the discipline of hope in a time that can feel quite hopeless. How to create change in a healthcare system that seems like it does. not. want. to. change.

Instead, it developed as a more ethereal story, one about patterns.

The more I looked at the intersection of art and med-icine, the more connected it became. It is astounding that the first recorded physician in ancient Egypt, Imhotep, was also an architect and "Chief Sculptor, and Maker of Vases in Chief."[1] How about that iron-rich ochre, which is featured in the color palette of this book, has been used for more than 100,000 years as a sun protectant, antibacterial, and medicinal salve as well as in paint? Or that sound, which is considered "one of the oldest tools in medicine,"[2] is crucial to diagnostic technologies today and even emerging in neurology as a treatment for depression and epilepsy?[3] It's all so beautiful.

By collaborating with artists and thinking like an artist myself for this book, I became more curious than mad about healthcare (curious is vastly more useful than mad). That curiosity helped me realize that many of the problems that feel impossible are actually quite new. We're only about 100 years into the seismic shift that rapidly reformed Western medicine as a hard science in reaction to a new understanding of germs and bacteria — a shift that delivered us breathtaking progress and lives saved but also maybe left healthcare literally sanitized, for better and worse.

The white coats, the systems of education and credentialing, the culture of medicine, the insurance companies and hospitals, the sounds of ICU alarms, the colors of latex gloves — these are all things people decided, and usually not all that long ago. The status quo would gladly have you think that it is all carved into stone, Hippocrates himself dictating ICD-10 codes. Instead, it is as transient as the lines tracing across EKG paper. It's ethereal, and it's powerful to imagine all the ways medicine could be shifted again 100 years from now.

My hope is for that shift to bring art and medicine back together, closer and in abundance again. In quantum entanglement, it is observed that two particles, once linked together, will stay bonded — reacting together even when physically miles apart. After this book, art and medicine seem entangled in that way. Sometimes wandering, yet always connected across space and time.

What happens when we help art and medicine be together again? In these chapters, we've seen that it could look like listening more to patients, to communities, to colleagues, to our past, to our imaginations for what is next. The future could be more playful, more colorful, more curious about new ways. It could help us forgive the harm done and forgive ourselves for, of course, not being able to fix everything all on our own. It could bring us together to heal. This is the work of remaking medicine. Can you imagine it?

END

Index

Citations

PROLOGUE

Narrative sources:
1. Mirror, Mirror 2021: Reflecting Poorly: Health Care in the U.S. Compared to Other High-Income Countries. (2021). *Commonwealth Fund.* commonwealthfund.org.
2. Demoralized. (n.d.). In C. McIntosh (Ed.), *Cambridge Advanced Learner's Dictionary & Thesaurus.* Cambridge University Press.
3. Kidder, T. (2003). *Mountains Beyond Mountains: The Quest of Dr. Paul Farmer, A Man Who Would Cure the World.* Random House.
4. Walter, D. (2020). The remarkable Neal Stephenson interview. *Damien Walter.* damiengwalter.com.

TIME

1.1 HISTORIC ABUNDANCE
Narrative sources:
1. Lovejoy, B. (2016). A Brief History of Medical Cannibalism. *Lapham's Quarterly.* laphamsquarterly.org.
2. Evil Spirits as a Cause of Sickness in Babylonia. (1905). *Nature,* 71, 249–250.
3. Miller, L. J. (2017). Divine Punishment or Disease? Medieval and Early Modern Approaches to the 1518 Strasbourg Dancing Plague. *Dance Research, (2),* 149–164.
4. Tognotti, E. (2013). *Lessons from the History of Quarantine, from Plague to Influenza A. Emerging Infectious Diseases, (2),* 254–259.
5. Langwick, S. A. (2011). *Bodies, Politics, and African Healing* (pp. 8,22). Indiana University Press.
6. Fancourt, D. (2017). A history of the use of arts in health. *Oxford Academic.*
7. Sooke, A. (2014). Leonardo da Vinci's groundbreaking anatomical sketches. *BBC Culture.* bbc.com

8. Dahan, S., & Shoenfeld, Y. (2017). *A Picture is Worth a Thousand Words: Art and Medicine. The Israel Medical Association Journal, 19* (12), 772–776.
9. Clayton, M. (2012). Medicine: Leonardo's anatomy years. *Nature, (7394),* 314–316.
10. National Library of Medicine. (2011). *Islamic Culture and the Medical Arts: Anatomy.* (Original work published 1994). nlm.nih.gov.
11. Vesalius, A. (1555). *De Humani Corporis Fabrica.* Johann Oporinus.
12. Simon, J., Chadwick, A., & Craker, L. (1984). *Herbs: An Indexed Bibliography 1971-1980 the Scientific Literature on Selected Herbs, and Aromatic and Medicinal Plants of the Temperate Zone.* Archon Books.
13. Semwal, R. B., Semwal, D. K., Combrinck, S., Cartwright-Jones, C., & Viljoen, A. (2014). *Lawsonia inermis L. (henna): Ethnobotanical, phytochemical and pharmacological aspects. Journal of Ethnopharmacology, (1),* 80–103.
14. Mahmood, Z. A., Zoha, S. M., Usmanghani, K., Hasan, M. M., Ali, O., Jahan, S., Saeed, A., Zaihd, R., & Zubair, M. (2009). Kohl (surma): retrospect and prospect. *Pakistan Journal of Pharmaceutical Sciences, 22* (1), 107–122.
15. Quarcoopome, N. O., Richardson, J., & Elaine L. (2012). When Art Works (p. 4). Wayne State University. art.wayne.edu.
16. The 5 Elements of African art are used to describe the aesthetics. (2017). *Black Art Story.* blackartstory.org.
17. Murrell, D. (2008). African Influences in Modern Art. The Metropolitan Museum of Art. metmuseum.org.
18. Slave Medicine. (n.d.). Thomas Jefferson's Monticello. monticello.org.
19. Rothman, D. J., Marcus, S., & Kiceluk, S. A. (1995). *Medicine and Western Civilization* (pp. 343, 348, 376–379). Rutgers University Press.

20. Goodman, J., McElligott, A., & Marks, L. (2004). Useful Bodies (p. 2). Johns Hopkins University Press.

21. Relman, A. S. (1980). The New Medical-Industrial Complex. *New England Journal of Medicine, (17),* 963–970.

22. Schneider, E. C., Sarnak, D. O., Squires, D., Shah, A., & Doty, M. M. (2017). Mirror, mirror 2017: international comparison reflects flaws and opportunities for better health care. The Commonwealth Fund. commonwealthfund.org.

23. Costello, J. (2016). Enhancing visual acuity in medical education through the arts. Artstor. artstor.org.

24. Fancourt, D. & Finn, S. (2019). *What Is the Evidence on the Role of the Arts in Improving Health and Well-Being.* World Health Organization. apps.who.int.

25. Fancourt, D. (2017). *A history of the use of arts in health.* Oxford University Press.

26. Courtney, C. A., O'Hearn, M. A., & Franck, C. C. (2016). Frida Kahlo: Portrait of Chronic Pain. *Physical Therapy, 97 (1),* 90-96.

27. Lorde, A. (2020). *The Cancer Journals.* Penguin.

28. Charon, R. (2001). Narrative Medicine. *JAMA, (15).*

29. Epstein, R. M. & Street, R. L. (2011). The Values and Value of Patient-Centered Care. *The Annals of Family Medicine,* 9 (2), 100–103.

30. Poulos, R. G., Marwood, S., Harkin, D., Opher, S., Clift, S., Cole, A., ... Poulos, C. J. (2018). Arts on prescription for community-dwelling older people with a range of health and wellness needs. *Health Social Care in the Community, (2),* 483–492.

31. Rollins, J., Sonke, J., Cohen, R., Boles, A., & Li, J. (2009). *State of the field report: Arts in healthcare 2009.* Society for the Arts in Healthcare. americansforthearts.org.

32. Bungay, H. & Clift, S. (2010). Arts on Prescription: A review of practice in the UK. *Perspectives in Public Health,* 130 (6), 277–281.

Images:

1. *Venus of Willendorf* [Photograph]. (n.d.). Bradshaw Foundation. bradshawfoundation.com.

1.2 LOOKING BACK

Artwork (commissioned from James Lee Chiahan):

1. Chiahan, J. L. (2022). *Past* [Illustration].

Narrative sources:

1. Weber, Bruce. (2013). Jane Wright, Oncology Pioneer, Dies at 93. *The New York Times.* nytimes.com.

2. Celebrating Black History Month: A Profile on the Pioneering Dr. Jane Cooke Wright. (2022). *Physicians Committee for Responsible Medicine.* pcrm.org.

1.4 BOUNDARY SAINTS

1. Two legacies of caring—one ministry of change. (n.d.). *CommonSpirit.* commonspirit.org.

2. Our Heritage: How We Began. (n.d.). *Providence.* providence.org.

3. Friedmann, Jonathan, L. (2020). *Jewish Los Angeles* (p. 1913). Arcadia Publishing.

4. Stulberg, D. B., Lawrence, R. E., Shattuck, J., & Curlin, F. A. (2010). Religious Hospitals and Primary Care Physicians: Conflicts over Policies for Patient Care. *Journal of General Internal Medicine, (7),* 725–730.

5. Solomon, T., Uttley, L., Hasbrouck, P., & Jung, Y. (2020). Bigger and Bigger – The Growth of Catholic Health Systems. *Community Catalyst.* communitycatalyst.org.

6. Koenig, H. G. (2000). Religion and Medicine I: Historical Background and Reasons for Separation. *The International Journal of Psychiatry in Medicine*, (4), 385–398.
7. Proudfoot, W. & Shaver, P. R. (1997). Attribution Theory and the Psychology of Religion. In B. Spilka & D. N. McIntosh (Eds.), *The Psychology Of Religion* (p. 139). Routledge.
8. Hefner, R. (2003). [From a lecture at Boston University].
9. McDougall, H. (2011). St Francis of Assisi: a saint for our times. *The Guardian*. theguardian.com
10. Carroll, L. (2019). Patients don't care about provider religious ties, expect all needed care. *Reuters*. reuters.com
11. Crist, C. (2019). Many Catholic hospitals fail to disclose religious affiliation, restrictions online. *Reuters*. reuters.com
12. Sack, K. (2011). Nuns, a 'Dying Breed,' Fade From Leadership Roles at Catholic Hospitals. *The New York Times*. nytimes.com
13. Schlosberg, J., Griswold, L., Yamada, H., McDonald, J., & Osunsami, S. (2022). America's nun population in steep decline. *ABC News*. abcnews.go.com.
14. King, R. (2021). Nonprofit hospitals spend less on charity care than for-profits, study finds. *Fierce Healthcare*. fiercehealthcare. com.
15. Pattison, M. (2021). Hidden costs: When for-profit chains buy Catholic hospitals. *Crux*. cruxnow.com.
16. Berg, N. (2011). Why Does California's Central Valley Have Such Bad Air Pollution? *Bloomberg*. bloomberg.com.
17. Dangberg, L. C. (2021). UC, Catholic health care partnership is saving lives. *San Francisco Examiner*. sfexaminer.com.

BODY

2.1 ACTS OF CARE

Narrative sources:

1. Expressions: A body of work. (2012). *Scrubs Magazine*. scrubsmag.com.
2. Weatherspoon Art Museum Uncg. (2021). *Weatherspoon Art Museum Conversation with Artist Nate Lewis for Art on Paper 2021*. YouTube. youtube.com.

Images (all licensed from Nate Lewis):

1. Lewis, N. (2020). *Probing the Land V* [Artwork].
2. Lewis, N. (2015). *Still Symphony* [Artwork].
3. Lewis, N. (2021). *Orchestra in the Valley* [Artwork].

2.2 MOVING PERSPECTIVES

Narrative sources:

1. Tsaplina, M. (2020). Bodies speaking: Embodiment, illness and the poetic materiality of puppetry/object practice. *Journal of Applied Arts & Health, 11* (1 & 2), 85–102.
2. Re-Imagining Medicine. (n.d.). *The Kenan Institute for Ethics*. kenan.ethics.duke.edu.
3. Tsaplina, M. (2021). Animate Earth-Dream Puppet, the poetic knowledges of ancient forests and disabled communities. *Orion Magazine*. orionmagazine.org.
4. Kanngieser, A. & Todd, Z. (2021). Listening as Relation, an Invocation. *AM Kanngieser*. amkanngieser.com.

Images (all shared by Marina Tsapalina):

1. Zimmerman, R. (2018). [Four students from Duke University's *Reimagine Medicine* cohort engaging in an *Embodiment, Disability, and Puppetry* training holding a bulky, water-stone-like puppet with diverse limb attachments made by Marina Tsaplina and Torry Bend.]

2. Zimmerman, R. (2018). [Three students from Duke University's *Reimagine Medicine* cohort engaging in an *Embodiment, Disability, and Puppetry* training holding a square-bodied, rose-blooming puppet with heart-caged feet made by Marina Tsaplina and Torry Bend.]

SIGHT

3.1 ON BEING SEEN
Images (all licensed from Kathleen Sheffer):
1. Sheffer, K. (2017). [Photograph of a dated, torn fluid intake and output catalog meticulously handwritten by the patient in the hospital].
2. Sheffer, K. (2016). [Self-portrait of Kathleen with fresh chest scars taken in hospital mirror 20 days post-op. Photographer looks down and away].
3. Sheffer, K. (2016). [Image of a typed description of Kathleen's transplant procedure].
4. Sheffer, K. (2017). [Self-portrait of Kathleen with healed chest scars taken in bathroom mirror 245 days post-op. Photographer stares straight ahead].
5. Sheffer, K. (2016). [Self-portrait of Kathleen with chest scars obscured by paper cranes drawn with henna ink. Mother smiles in the background while sister brushes teeth].
6. Sheffer, K. (2017). *Double-Lung Transplant 5.1.08* [Black and white photograph of a double-lung transplant survivor showing scars].
7. Sheffer, K. (2017) *Heart Transplant 2.3.16* [Black and white photograph of a heart transplant survivor showing scars].

3.2 ON SEEING
Images (all licensed from Dr. Syed T. Hoda):
1. Hoda. S. T. (n.d.). *Coupled* [Photograph].

2. Hoda. S. T. (n.d.). *Viewed* [Photograph].
3. Hoda. S. T. (n.d.). *Traffic* [Photograph].

SPACE

4.1 BUILDING DIGNITY
Narrative sources:
1. Kinney, J. (2016). Architect Talks Design as an Engine for Healing and Change. *Next City*. nextcity.org.
2. Murphy, M. P. & Mansfield, J. (2021). *The Architecture of Health: Hospital Design and the Construction of Dignity* (p. 12). Cooper Hewitt, Smithsonian Design Museum.

Images (shared by MASS Design Group):
1. MASS Design Group. (n.d.). [Photograph of Butaro District Hospital roof and surrounding area].
2. MASS Design Group. (n.d.). [Photograph of plants outside of Butaro District Hospital].
3. MASS Design Group. (n.d.). [Photograph of two women walking in an outdoor corridor of Butaro District Hospital].
4. Baan, I. (n.d.). [Photograph of people seated outside of Butaro District Hospital].

4.2 REASSEMBLY
Narrative sources:
1. Superarchitecture 1966-1968. (n.d.). *Cristiano Toraldo di Francia*. cristiano-toraldodifrancia.it.
2. Wallis, S. (2016). A '60s Architecture Collective That Made History (but No Buildings). *The New York Times*. nytimes.com.
3. Imam, J. (2021). Architects Dreaming of a Future With No Buildings. *The New York Times*. nytimes.com.

4. Cristina, M. (2017). *SuperDesign: Italian Radical Design 1965-75*. The Monacelli Press.

5. Adolfo Natalini, Cristiano Toraldo di Francia, et al. (1982). *Superstudio & Radicals* (p. 224). Japan Interior.

6. Chiappone-Piriou, E., Migayrou, F., Lampariello, B., Mastrigli, G., & Fujii, H. (2021). *Superstudio Migrazioni* (p. 21). Walther König.

Image/artwork (commissioned from Dr. Laura J. Tafe):

1. Tafe, L. (2022). *Big Data* [Analog collage].

2. Tafe, L. (2022). *Compassion* [Analog collage].

3. Tafe, L. (2022). *Community* [Analog collage].

4. Tafe, L. (2022). *Personhood* [Analog collage].

SOUND

5.1 TONE SHIFT

Narrative sources:

1. Cho, O. M., Kim, H., Lee, Y. W., & Cho, I. (2016). *Clinical Alarms in Intensive Care Units: Perceived Obstacles of Alarm Management and Alarm Fatigue in Nurses. Healthcare informatics research, 22* (1), 46–53.

2. TEDMED. (2019). *How one musician is reimagining hospital sounds*. YouTube. youtube.com.

3. Sen, Y. Biography. *Yoko K.* yoko.mu.

4. Sen, Y. (2015). IDEO Cambridge Fortnight | The Mother Tongue by Ayyoko Confidential. Vimeo. vimeo.com.

5. Patient safety. (2019, March 9). World Health Organization. who.int.

6. Joseph, B. & Joseph, M. (2016). The health of the healthcare workers. *Indian Journal of Occupational and Environmental Medicine, 20* (2), 71–72.

Artwork (commissioned from James Lee Chiahan):

1. Chiahan, J. L. (2022). *Tone Shift* [Illustration].

COLOR

6.1 THE CHROMA PROJECT

Narrative sources:

1. Mironidou-Tzouveleki, M. & Tzitzis, P. (2014). *Medical practice in the ancient Asclepeion in Kos island. Hellenic Journal of Nuclear Medicine, 17* (3), 167-70.

2. Stefanini, S. & Sasdelli, G. (2015). Asclepeion of Kos. *Himetop.* himetop. wikidot.com

3. Murphy, M. P. & Mansfield, J. (2021). *The Architecture of Health: Hospital Design and the Construction of Dignity* (p. 40). Cooper Hewitt, Smithsonian Design Museum.

4. History of Sant Pau Hospital. *Sant Pau Recinte Modernista.* santpaubarcelona.org.

5. Birren, F. (1955). *New Horizons in Color.* Reinhold Publishing.

6. Saxon, W. (1988). Faber Birren, 88, Expert on Color. *The New York Times.*

7. Birren, F. (1950). *Color Psychology and Color Therapy.* McGraw-Hill.

8. Nightingale, F. (1969). *Notes on Nursing: What It Is, and What It Is Not.* Dover Publications.

9. Rosenberg, A. R., Orellana, L., Wolfe, J., & Dussel, V. (2018). *The Limitations of "How Are You Feeling?" Journal of Pain and Symptom Management,* (3), e6–e8.

Images (commissioned from Anna Engstrom):

1. Engstrom, A. (2022). [Image of an orange badge on orange background].

2. Engstrom, A. (2022). [Image of a female patient wearing an orange badge].

3. Engstrom, A. (2022). [Image of a female patient with a badge conversing with a provider].

4. Engstrom, A. (2022). [Image of a female patient choosing badge color from an orange wall].

5. Engstrom, A. (2022). [Image of patients in a hospital lobby beside an interactive digital canvas wall].

6. Engstrom, A. (2022). [Image of people standing outside of a hospital with a colorful wall].

Stock images used and modified for the purpose of the artwork concepts:

1. Mueses, J. (2018). *Photo of Five Cars Parked* [Photograph]. Pexels. pexels.com

2. Roma, A. (2021). *Millennial Woman Looking into Distance on Sunny Day* [Photograph]. Pexels. pexels.com

3. Anaday, A. (2019). *HD Photo by Abby Anaday* [Photograph]. Unsplash. unsplash.com.

4. Anne, K. (2018). *Three Woman Holding Hands While Walking Photo* [Photograph]. Unsplash. unsplash.com.

5. Bennett, L. (2018). *Three Green-Leafed Plants* [Photograph]. Unsplash. unsplash.com.

6. Botta, V. (2017). *White Armless Chair near White Wall Photo* [Photograph]. Unsplash. unsplash.com.

7. Châtel-Innocenti, P. (2017). *White Pendant Lamp Photo* [Photograph]. Unsplash. unsplash.com.

8. *Doctor Full Length Portrait Stock Photo* [Photograph]. (2015). Alamy. alamy.com.

9. Pimkina, D. (2020). *HD Photo by Daria Pimkina* [Photograph]. Unsplash. unsplash.com.

10. Rasmussen, K. (2018). *Man Standing under Building Photo* [Photograph]. Unsplash. unsplash.com.

11. Rawson-Harris, J. (2018). *Woman Standing beside Shelf Photo* [Photograph]. Unsplash. unsplash.com.

12. Ruttan, G. (2020). *White and Brown Concrete Building under Blue Sky during Daytime Photo* [Photograph]. Unsplash. unsplash.com.

13. Stecanella, G. (2019). *Woman Standing on Ice Photo* [Photograph]. Unsplash. unsplash.com.

14. Vázquez, D. (2018). *Photo of Cannabis Plant with Pot Photo* [Photograph]. Unsplash. unsplash.com.

15. Hazzan, H., Burton, R., Pearson, C., Suzuki, H., & Melluso, D. (2019). Adapted from *Doctor Using Stethoscope to Examine a Woman* [Photograph]. Flickr. flickr.com. CC BY 4.0.

16. Hazzan, H., Burton, R., Pearson, C., Suzuki, H., & Melluso, D. (2019). Adapted from *Doctor with Vaccine Tray Talking to a Young Woman* [Photograph]. Flickr. flickr.com. CC BY 4.0.

6.2 PATHOLOGY OF MEDICAL COLORS
Narrative sources:

1. How Can I Recycle (or Upcycle) Empty Prescription Pill Bottles? (2021). *GoodRx*. goodrx.com.

2. Sabanoglu, T. (2021). Total number of retail prescriptions filled annually in the U.S. 2013-2025. *Statista*. statista.com.

3. In the Courts: Johnson & Johnson vs the American Red Cross. (2008). *WIPO Magazine*. wipo.int.

4. Red Cross. (2021). *History.com*. history.com.

5. Dsouza, O., Shetty, A., & Shetty S. (2014). Medical Symbols in Practice: Myths vs

Reality. *Journal of Clinical and Diagnostic Research, 8* (8), PC12-PC14.

6. The Story Behind BAND-AID® Brand. (1964). *The Kiplinger Magazine,* 32.

7. BAND-AID® [@bandaidbrand]. (2020). *We hear you. We see you...* [Photograph]. Instagram. instagram.com

8. Medical, Nursing, Hospital, Surgery & Home Health Supplies. (n.d.). *Medegen Medical Company.* medegenmed.com.

9. Garber, M. (2018). 20 Years of Viagra. *The Atlantic.* theatlantic.com.

10. Mukherjee, S. (2018). Viagra Anniversary: How Much Pfizer Has Made off the Drug. *Fortune.* fortune.com.

11. Epic UserWeb Sign In. (n.d.). *Epic.* epic.com.

12. About Us. (n.d.). *Epic.* epic.com.

13. Sherman, H. (1914). The Green Operating Room at St. Luke's Hospital. *California State Journal of Medicine, 12* (5), 181–183.

14. Ensign, J. (2015). The Color of Hospitals. *Josephine Ensign.* josephineensign.com.

15. Pantalony, D. (2009). The colour of medicine. *Canadian Medical Association Journal, 181* (6-7), 402-403.

16. Fact check: Two-tone medical masks should be worn with color side facing out. (2020). *Reuters.* reuters.com.

17. Sibbald, B. (2002). Hospitals leaving huge "ecological footprints": report. *Canadian Medical Association Journal, 166* (3), 363.

18. Hohti, P. (2019). Exploring Historical Blacks: The Burgundian Black Collaboratory. *Refashioning the Renaissance.* refashioningrenaissance.eu.

19. Hochberg, M. (2007). The Doctor's White Coat: An Historical Perspective. AMA *Journal of Ethics, 9* (4), 310-314.

20. Harrah, S. (2021). The White Coat Ceremony – A Rich Tradition For Medical Students. *University of Medicine and Health Sciences.* umhs-sk.org.

DREAMS

7.1 RESTORATIVE

Narrative sources:

1. Sarkar, D., Walker-Swaney, J., & Shetty, K. (2019). Food Diversity and Indigenous Food Systems to Combat Diet-Linked Chronic Diseases. *Current developments in nutrition, 4* (Suppl 1), 3–11.

2. Hatala, A. R., Njeze, C., Morton, D., Pearl, T., & Bird-Naytowhow, K. (2020). Land and nature as sources of health and resilience among Indigenous youth in an urban Canadian context: a photovoice exploration. *BMC public health, 20* (1), 538.

3. Intergovernmental Panel on Climate Change. (2016). *Special Report on Climate Change and Land.* Chapter 3: Desertification.

4. United States Environmental Protection Agency. (2022). *Navajo Nation: Cleaning Up Abandoned Uranium Mines.* epa.gov.

5. Center for Native Environmental Health Equity Research. (n.d.). UNM Health Sciences Center. hsc.unm.edu.

6. Indian Health Service. (2019). *Indian Health Disparities Fact Sheet.* ihs.gov.

7. Gone, J. P. & Trimble, J. E. (2012). American Indian and Alaska Native mental health: diverse perspectives on enduring disparities. *Annual review of clinical psychology, 8,* 131–160.

Images (all licensed from April Bojorquez from DesertArtLAB):

1. DesertArtLAB. (n.d.). [Photograph of children and a woman surrounded by cactus plants].

2. DesertArtLAB. (n.d.). [Photograph of children outside preparing food by a cart].

3. DesertArtLAB. (n.d.). [Photograph of a front-loader tricycle displayed in an art gallery].

7.2 A PUBLIC HOME

Artwork (commissioned from Fernando Martí):

1. Martí, F. (2022). [Artwork].

7.3 DREAMSPACE

Narrative sources:

1. Norris, J. (2022). How does space travel impact the human brain? *Medical News Today*. medicalnewstoday.com.
2. Foust, J. (2022). Entire NASA astronaut corps eligible for Artemis missions. *Space News*. spacenews.com.
3. Hock, D. (Producer) & Mader, J (Director). (2022). *Space Health: Surviving In The Final Frontier*. Translational Research Institute for Space Health. spacehealth-themovie.com.
4. BEYOND: An Art Experience that immerses audiences in underrepresented perspec-tives on climate change at COP26. (n.d.). *Google Arts & Culture*. artsandculture. google.com.
5. St. Jude patients guide Inspiration4 astro-nauts via Voices of Inspiration immersive digital experience. (2021). *PR Newswire*. prnewswire.com.
6. Refik Anadol: An Important Memory for Humanity NFT Artwork Collection. (2022). *Creative Work Studios*. creativeworkstu-dios.com.

Images:

1. Space for Art Foundation. (2021). [Photograph of the BEYOND Art Spacesuit at COP26]
2. Z3VR. (n.d.). [Image of virtual reality program tower lobby].
3. Z3VR. (n.d.). [Image of virtual reality program portal].

ACTION

8.1 PAPERWEIGHT

Narrative sources:

1. Otis Gallery LLC. (2021). *Post-Qualification Offering Statement Amendment No. 23* (File No. 024-10951). United States Securities and Exchange Commission. sec.gov.
2. Health Care Debt In The U.S.: The Broad Consequences Of Medical And Dental Bills. (2022). *Kaiser Family Foundation*. kff.org.
3. Himmelstein, D., Thorne, D., Warren, E., & Woolhandler, S. (2009). Medical Bankruptcy in the United States, 2007: Results of a National Study. *The American Journal of Medicine, 122* (8), (741-746).
4. Anderson, G. F., Hussey, P., & Petrosyan, V. (2019). It's Still The Prices, Stupid: Why The US Spends So Much On Health Care, And A Tribute To Uwe Reinhardt. *Health Affairs,* (1), 87–95.
5. Charles, S. (2021). What the rise of GoFundMe's to pay medical bills says about US health care system. *The Grio*. thegrio.com.
6. Igra, M. & Kenworthy, N. (2021). Medical Crowdfunding and Disparities in Health Care Access in the United States, 2016-2020. *American Journal of Public Health, 112,* (491-498).
7. Dollar For, [@dollarfor]. (2021). *#stitch with @420loveontour hospital bills are lame. Let's take care of em! #fyp #legal #medicalbills*. [Video]. TikTok. tiktok.com.
8. Weissmann, D. (2021). The Medical-bill "Negotiation Lab." *In An Arm and a Leg*. armandalegshow.com.
9. Noguchi, Y. (2022). This group's wiped out $6.7 billion in medical debt, and it's just getting started. *NPR*. npr.org.

Images:
1.   MSCHF. (2020). *$8,603.45 of 3 Medical Bills* [Artwork].

8.3 LOOKING AHEAD
Artwork (commissioned from James Lee Chiahan):
1.   Chiahan, J. L. (2022). *Future* [Illustration].

Narrative sources:
1.   About Foldit. (n.d.). *Foldit*. fold.it.

8.4 INSIDE JOB
Narrative sources:
1.   With Mettle Health, BJ Miller and Sonya Dolan Seek to 'Bring Intention & Creativity to the Experience of Dying.' (2021). *Enjoy Mill Valley*. enjoymillvalley.com.
2.   Forshee, Z., Manceor, C., & McGinness, R. (2022). Your Artistry and Values. In V. Hartman, K. DeLaurenti, & S. Thomas (Eds.), *The Path to Funding: The Artist's Guide to Building Your Audience, Generating Income, and Realizing Career Sustainability.* The Peabody Institute of The Johns Hopkins University.

EPILOGUE

Narrative sources:
1.   Aaltonen, G. (2013). *The History of Architecture: Iconic Buildings Throughout the Ages.* Arcturus Publishing.
2.   Babikian, T., Zeltzer, L., Tachdjian, V., Henry L., Javanfard, E., Tucci, L., Gooddarzi, M., & Tachdjian, R. (2013). Music as Medicine: A Review and Historical Perspective. *Mary Ann Liebert, Inc.* liebertpub.com.
3.   Kubanek, J., Ye, J. B., Moore, K. B. P., & Newsome, W. (2020). Remote, brain region–specific control of choice behavior with ultrasonic waves. *Science Advances.* science.org.

COLOPHON

Narrative sources:
1.   Fayerman, P. (2012). What do blooming snowdrops have to do with Alzheimer's disease treatment and Homer's Odyssey? *Vancouver Sun.*
2.   Moed, L., Shwayder, T. A., & Chang, M. W. (2001). Cantharidin Revisited: A Blistering Defense of an Ancient Medicine. *JAMA.*

Biographies

In order of appearance

emilyfpeters.com
@emilyfpeters

EMILY F. PETERS is the founder and CEO of the healthcare brand strategy studio, Uncommon Bold, and creative director of Procedure Press. In 2016, she survived a near-fatal amniotic fluid embolism in childbirth and became an advocate for blood donation. She lives in San Francisco with her husband, daughter, and pink poodle, Benny.

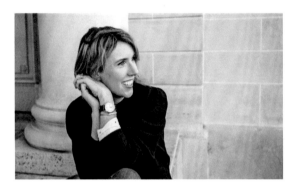

kelliemenendez.com
@kelliesf7

KELLIE MENENDEZ is an artist, mother, founder, dancer, designer, and investor. Menendez founded Half Full in 2015 as a culmination of her passion for the wild world and her desire to create beauty. Half Full's celebrated patterns on wallpapers and textiles have reached thousands while also giving back to causes that heal our planet.

@rootsofresistance

SADE MUSA draws from a background in biomedical research, western herbalism, and African-American folk medicine. Musa founded Roots of Resistance — a project that seeks to reconnect people with their ancestral healing practices, disrupt colonial narratives invisibilizing Afro-diasporic contributions to medicine, and address health inequity through the provision of accessible wellness education and services. Roots of Resistance operates under the belief that bodily autonomy and culturally relevant medical care are essential and that learning to heal ourselves is a liberatory praxis of self-determination and resistance.

jlee.ca
@buttmcbutt

JAMES LEE CHIAHAN is a Taiwanese-Canadian artist currently working out of Montreal, Canada. He is interested in expressing different moments and memories in time with some underlying, inexplicable color of what it feels like to be alive and to be living simultaneously in the past and in the present. Currently, he is exploring the ideas of impermanence, loss, fear, and the mercurial nature of memory and experience.

sandeepjauhar.com
@sandeepjauhar

SANDEEP JAUHAR, MD, PHD, is a practicing cardiologist at Northwell Health. He is the author of three bestselling books: *Intern: A Doctor's Initiation, Doctored: The Disillusionment of an American Physician,* and *Heart: A History.* His latest book is *My Father's Brain: Life in the Shadow of Alzheimer's.* Dr. Jauhar is a frequent contributor to The New York Times, and his essays have also been published in *The Wall Street Journal, Time,* and *Slate.*

@jonathonfeit

JONATHON S. FEIT, MBA, MA, is co-founder and CEO of Beyond Lucid Technologies, an award-winning health-and-safety innovations firm that connects fire and EMS agencies with hospitals and public health services and powers America's first statewide registry of children with special health needs. He holds advanced degrees from Carnegie Mellon and Boston University and graduate certificates from MIT Sloan and Pepperdine Caruso School of Law. Feit has Tourette's Syndrome and advocates passionately on behalf of people with disabilities. In 2022, he received a Civilian EMS Award from the State of California.

"For my extraordinary parents, Harold and Brenda, who first taught me to venture into the world, then taught me to constantly question it, and inexplicably found faith enough to never hesitate in helping me try to impact it. And for my teachers — Lisa Suennen ("You only get what you ask for"), David Wolpe ("We have but one set of eyes"), and the late Geoffrey Hill, who would have agreed that words deserve both love and reverence, for at their nexus politics explode."

natelewisart.com
@nloois

NATE LEWIS began his career in healthcare working as a critical care nurse for nine years. He has had exhibitions and residencies throughout the country with organizations such as California African American Museum, The Yale Center for British Art, and Pioneer Works, showing pieces that draw from anatomy, physiology, and disease processes. Focusing on body representation, Lewis's work explores history through intricate patterns, textures, and rhythm, creating meditations of celebration, and lamentations.

marinatsaplina.com
@bodypoemspuppetry

MARINA "HERON" TSAPLINA is an eco-artist, educator, writer, independent scholar, and disability culture activist. As lead artist and co-founder of *Reimagine Medicine,* she was an associate of the Trent Center for Bioethics, Humanities & History of Medicine at Duke University (2018–2020). She holds a master's in bioethics and medical humanities, and was the strategy and action lead of NYinsulin4all with T1International (2019–2020). Currently, she is developing *Soil Spirit Forest,* a project in ancient, endangered, and disappeared forests that weaves ecological intimacy between human beings and the earth.

Marina Tsaplina thanks Dr. Jules Odendahl-James and Torry Bend for their collaboration and support for the development of the Embodiment, Disability, and Puppetry training in 2018, and Gair McCullough, program coordinator at Duke University.

ranaawdishmd.com
@ranaawdish

RANA AWDISH, MD, FCCP, is a critical care physician, pulmonologist, author of *In Shock,* and medical director of the Pulmonary Hypertension Program at Henry Ford Hospital. She is an advocate for connected care and serves as the Medical Director of Care Experience for Henry Ford Health, where she has integrated compassionate communication strategies and narrative medicine practice into the curriculum.

kathleensheffer.com
@kathleen.s.photography

KATHLEEN SHEFFER is a sought-after commercial and art photographer and advocate for transplant patients. Born with a heart condition and diagnosed with pulmonary hypertension, she developed a talent for photography early on in her patient journey. Only months after graduating from UC Berkeley and starting her photography business, Sheffer was listed for a heart-lung transplant. She got the call 28 days later and immediately turned her camera to herself — using photographs to be seen as more than just a patient.

With gratitude and admiration for all participants in the Scar Narratives project: Corie Crowe, Bradley Dell, Lindsay Garthwait, Leilani Graham, Mary Hazdovac, ToneeRose Legaspi, Mari Matsumura, and Kelly McCabe.

@01sth02

SYED T. HODA, MD, is a musician, photographer, writer, and physician. He is a director of Bone and Soft Tissue Pathology at NYU Langone Health and clinical associate professor at the NYU Grossman School of Medicine. He lives in Brooklyn, NYC, with his wife Sobia and seven-year-old son Emel, two cats, and too big a record collection for a small apartment.

@LJTafeMD

LAURA J. TAFE, MD, is a physician and collagist who works as an anatomic and molecular pathologist at Dartmouth Hitchcock Medical Center in Lebanon, New Hampshire. She has previously published analog collages in *Intima: A Journal of Narrative Medicine* and *Lifelines,* Geisel School of Medicine at Dartmouth Literary and art journal; had a collage selected as Cover Art, Honorable Mention, for the *Academic Medicine Journal*; and has shown her work in group shows at AVA Gallery and Art Center, also in Lebanon.

ambercooley.com
@ambercoolade

AMBER COOLEY is a brand researcher, coordinator, and music marketer. After studying marketing and music management at the University of the Pacific, Cooley embarked on a path to bridge the gap between creative expression and quantitative data through brand marketing. She now uses her love for music and ability to tell creative stories to help artists more effectively share their music with the world.

sydellerossmd.com
@sydellerossmd

SYDELLE ROSS, MD, D.ABA, grew up in the Republic of Trinidad and Tobago in the Caribbean telling her parents that she would someday become a singing doctor. Today, she is a triple board-certified anesthesiologist, pain specialist, and hospice and palliative medicine physician practicing with the U.S. Department of Veterans Affairs in New Jersey. Dr. Ross is also a classically trained soprano vocalist and host of the podcast *Prescriptions In Song* dedicated to promoting awareness of the healing potential of music.

tararajendran.com
@tara_rajendran

TARA RAJENDRAN, MBBS, MFA, was deemed a prodigy in the "saraswati veena," the national instrument of India, as a child. Her academic focus is hematological malignancies and music therapy in integrative oncology. Dr. Rajendran has presented her research at several national conferences and has attended hands-on clinical clerkships at Harvard Medical School, Weill Cornell, and Stanford Medicine. These clerkships inspired her to develop "Oncology & Strings," the first-ever lecture-concert music therapy-advocacy program.

annaengstromstudio.com
@anna.engstrom.studio

ANNA ENGSTROM is a color artist and design strategist leveraging human-centered design to solve complex healthcare challenges. Founder of AE Studio in San Francisco, she partners with companies and creative teams to envision, design, and build new experiences and ventures that raise the bar for women's health and contribute to greater gender equality — including IDEO, Tia Health, Evidation Health, CORA, Everlane, and Remind. Engstrom combines her human-centered design expertise with her abstract painting and her love for bold colors to reimagine brighter healthcare futures.

abakibeck.com
@winterweasel

ABAKI BECK, MPH, is a writer and public health doctoral student based in Minneapolis, Minnesota. She primarily writes about Indigenous science, knowledge, cultural revitalization, and gender-based violence in Native communities. In addition to writing, Beck has managed research projects to examine barriers and facilitators of healthcare access for low-income people, led program evaluation and reentry program design for a higher education in prison program, and assisted with health and Native American policy for a member of Congress. She is Blackfeet and Red River Métis.

@el_compay_nando

FERNANDO MARTÍ, M.ARCH, is a printmaker, writer, community architect, housing activist based in San Francisco, and a member of the Justseeds Artists' Cooperative. Martí's illustrations, etchings, linocuts, screenprints, public constructions, and altar ofrendas reflect his formal training in urbanism, his roots in rural Ecuador, and his current residence in the U.S. heart of Empire. His work reclaims ancestral traditions of place toward building a liberatory Latinx futurism in the city.

venturevalkyrie.com
@venturevalkyrie

LISA SUENNEN, MA, is the president of digital and data solutions at Canary Medical, Inc. and the CEO and managing partner of Venture Valkyrie, LLC. She has more than 30 years of experience in the healthcare field as an entrepreneur, venture capitalist, board member, and strategic advisor, and she is an internationally recognized author and speaker on healthcare, entrepreneurship, and venture capital topics. Suennen is also chair of the Scientific Advisory Board of the Translational Research Institute for Space Health (TRISH).

nickdawson.net
@nickpdawson

NICK DAWSON, MHA is the co-founder of the Emergency Design Collective and has led innovation at top healthcare organizations such as Kaiser Permanente, Johns Hopkins Medicine, and Bon Secours Health System. He has also advised the highest levels of the federal government, states, and localities on more human-centered health responses, working on big challenges that improve healthcare for patients, communities, and front-line providers.

@lisabari_threads

LISA BARI, MBA, MPH, is an American healthcare innovation executive. She is the CEO of Civitas Networks for Health, the national nonprofit organization with a mission to support community and data-led health improvement and information exchange to address health outcomes and provide the infrastructure for health equity. Bari previously served as the health IT and interoperability lead at the Centers for Medicare & Medicaid Services' Innovation Center and, earlier in her career, as a marketing executive for a primary care–focused health IT vendor.

justequityforhealth.com
@ammahstarr

STELLA SAFO, MD, MPH, is a Harvard-trained, board-certified HIV primary care physician; innovator in designing healthcare delivery models; founder of Just Equity for Health; and a founding member of Equity Now at Mount Sinai, Civic Health Alliance, and the Coalition to Advance Antiracism in Medicine. She continues practicing, teaching, researching, publishing, speaking to media, and exploring new opportunities for influence in pursuit of pushing medicine toward equity and justice.

| AUTHOR | Emily F. Peters |
| | emilyfpeters.com |

| CREATIVE PRODUCER | Joanne Lam |
| | joannelam.com |

PRODUCTION TEAM	Amber Cooley
	ambercooley.com
	Andrea Anguiano
	Ashley Greer
	ashleygreermedia.com
	Claudia Gutierrez-Smith
	Elaine Chen
	elainechen.info
	Linsey McNew
	linseymcnew.com
	Lucy Sansom
	Robert Peters
	rcpeters.com
	Sarah Stern
	sternsarah.com

| SPECIAL THANKS | Amanda Griffith, Kaitlin Rebella, Kina Mercado, Alison Meier, Sally Kim, Frances Baca, Sheila Cunningham, Setagaya Art Museum. |

PROCEDURE PRESS	An imprint of Uncommon Bold
	San Francisco, CA
	procedure.press
	@procedurepress

COLOPHON

Artist and textile designer Kellie Menendez created the repeating pattern of medicinal plants, both modern and ancient, for the endpapers of this book. Included are goji, coffee, California poppy, opium poppy, tamarind, and psilocybin mushroom. From daffodils and snowdrop bulbs, galantamine is used as a treatment for Alzheimer's disease[1] today and was mentioned in the ancient Greek epic poem, the *Odyssey,* as a medicine for reviving memory. Cantharidin from the blister beetle has also been used as medicine for more than 2,000 years in China and is still frequently applied in modern dermatology.[2] "Nature beautifully carries many secrets to healing and our own health — and reminds us that we're all part of these evolving systems on the planet," said Menendez.

The main body text of *Artists Remaking Medicine* is set to Jungka, a typeface developed collaboratively by Jungmyung Lee and Karel Martens from 2013 to 2015. Jungka shares the quality of a classically crafted sans serif typeface by taking formal cues from its historic predecessors Helvetica, Univers, and Akzidenz-Grotesk. With fine-tuned spacing for enhanced legibility, Jungka's accentuated circular curves evoke a soft, friendly, and rhythmical atmosphere with a modern touch.

Headings throughout the book are set to Bayard, a sans-serif typeface designed by Tré Seals of Vocal Type. Bayard is inspired by signs from the 1963 March On Washington For Jobs and Freedom, a political demonstration held in Washington, D.C., in 1963 by civil rights leaders to protest racial discrimination and to show support for major legislation that was pending in Congress. Bayard Rustin was appointed deputy director of the march, and in less than two months Rustin guided the organization of an event that would bring more than 200,000 participants to the nation's capital.

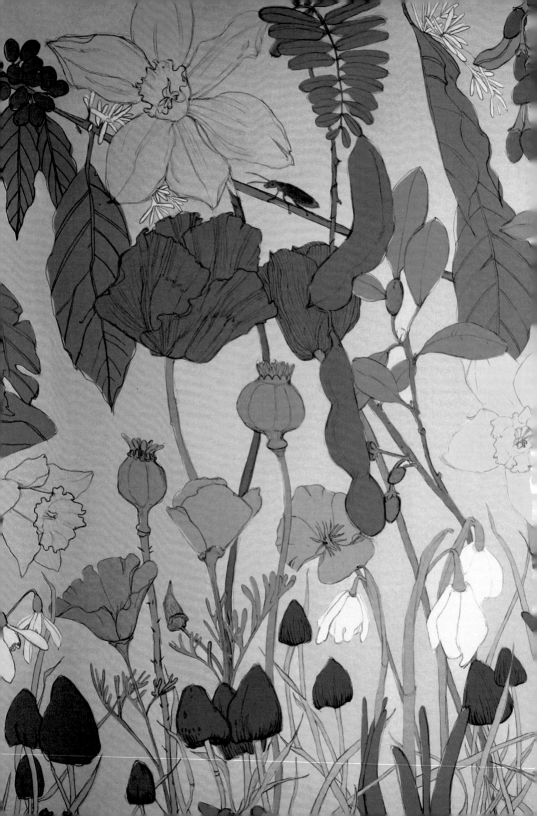